SOARING WITH CHRONIC ILLNESS

Live Your Best Life Everyday

Jennifer Bovee

About the Author:

Jennifer Bovee is a Licensed Clinical Social Worker passionate about empowering, mentoring, and inspiring her clients to believe in themselves and take charge of their lives and stories. Her impressive professional portfolio also includes designation and certification in Reciprocal Alcohol and Other Drug counseling, Clinical Trauma and Clinical Hypnotherapist, and Eye Movement Desensitization and Recovery therapy.

She is committed to being a positive influence in her clients' lives by helping them develop strong self-confidence and esteem in everything they set out to do. Jennifer firmly believes that our circumstances do not define us, and we have the power to rise above any obstacles we face and take control of our destinies. She treats all her clients like family with empathy, patience, and compassion. With over 25 years of experience in the field, Jennifer has honed her craft and gained invaluable customer service, communication, and problem-solving skills. She is committed to connecting with her clients and maintaining meaningful long-term relationships.

Jennifer is passionate about helping clients with terminal illnesses find and restore their physical, mental and emotional strength. She strives to develop and curate each experience to suit and cater to her client's unique situations and needs. Jennifer is reliable, kind, and passionate about spreading joy and happiness with her clients. She seeks to help people learn and develop healthy and positive habits and routines that contribute to their general well-being. Jennifer promises to be your guide, partner, and friend as you take on the journey to self-improvement and acceptance.

When she is not working, Jennifer enjoys spending quality time with her family friends and dog.

About the book:

It's about time you begin to feel heard even when no one is listening. To feel seen even when your illness is invisible to everyone.

Living with a chronic illness is no easy thing. It is often filled with a life of doubt, pain, dismissal from medical providers, accusations, and hopelessness. But it doesn't have to be that way.

Soaring With Chronic Illness offers practical advice, tips, and nuggets of encouragement from someone who has been in your shoes. Jenn Bovee, a trauma survivor, and chronic illness advocate, users her own debilitating experiences to offer a fresh, humorous take on what it's truly like living with chronic illnesses and one can do more than just manage it.

This book isn't written to suggest that you simply accept your body the way it is, like so many of our friends and physicians say. This book leaves you with something *deeper*, something *better*. A way for you to stop viewing your body as the enemy and start validating what you feel, see, and hear.

Reading this book will have you walking away with:

- **Actionable steps** to begin thriving in your chronic illness, rather than just surviving it
- The **encouragement** to view your body and mind with honor and self-love
- **Real stories** from the author to help you feel validated, seen, and heard
- The **strength to find your voice** so you can advocate for yourself

You do not have to walk in fear, disappointment, or silence any longer. *Soaring With Chronic Illness* is waiting to give you the tools and encouragement to not just survive, but thrive.

Table of Contents

CHAPTER 1

Life With A Chronic Illness

Have you ever felt betrayed or disappointed by a doctor or a physician? Can you recall that overall sense of benign hopelessness when dealing with the medical profession? I remember the sensation of laying on a cold metal table with a white sheet covering my face. I just wanted them to stop covering my face. Right now, I can't remember the exact words I tried to speak, but I assume it was something like, "hey, I'm awake" or, "uncover my face fools" (said like Mr. T of course), or something else equally argumentative at this point. What I most vividly remember is laying on that cold metal table, alone, just trying to figure out why they didn't respond to me. The depths of the betrayal that I was experiencing while lying there, trapped in an endless cycle of trauma and victimization, were inconceivable. The most mind-shattering part was being forced to just lay there, not being able to tell them that I was awake, not being able to will my body into movement, not being able to get their attention, just being completely and utterly powerless. Add to that the arrogant surgeon who had previously professed that, after this surgery, I would have no pain because he was "that good." And yet, here I was, feeling every pull, every tear, every stretch, every yank, every cut, and every incision.

Then it occurred to me that I had not gotten my voice to work. I was incapable of speech. It was like one of those horror movies where you see a woman on screen just trapped on the table, and they're doing surgery, but she is wide awake. That was what was occurring to me, to my own body!

When I finally got my voice to work, it was like something out of a bad mushroom trip, or at least what I imagine that must be like. I remember speaking my words clearly and enunciating properly but also be aware that my words were not coming out of my mouth the way I was saying them in my head. Had I had a stroke?! Was I dying?! Was I doing the dying talk people do before they die!? They still did not remove this sheet. Was I already dead!? Not again, please!!

I remember hearing the surgeon say, "Why is she talking? Someone shut her up!" My understanding is that they just tried to put me back under sedation. Only there were two major problems with this; the first one is that the original sedation did not take, and the second one was that I was feeling every cut and insertion they were performing for this surgery.

Because I am a trauma survivor, I did what I knew how to do. I stopped trying to talk, and I got very silent. I listened to that surgeon say the most horrible things about me.

If this story had any sort of happy conclusion, I would tell you that they wheeled me into a recovery area and drugged me up to the point that I visited Puff the Magic Dragon and dreamed of the land of Galilea. However, I imagine you're sensing a theme here, right? They skipped the recovery room and wheeled me back to the room where I'd started.

While they were wheeling me down the hall, I remember hearing someone ask the anesthesiologist why I wouldn't stop crying. When I recall hearing, her asking the question, the condescension and judgment are still so painful even now, years after it happened. She was not curious, it was just a straight-up judgment, "Why won't she stop crying?!" There was no attempt at comprehension or any care to explore what might have happened or have gone wrong.

It is important to note that not once during this process did anyone ever talk to me, check in on me, or even ask if I was okay. It seems like some amount of human decency is missing there, right? In hindsight, I suspect I passed out from the pain right after hearing the anesthesiologist tell the second person who'd complained about my crying to take me to my husband because that would probably, "shut me up."

When I'd met with the surgeon before the surgery and specifically reviewed the medications I was taking, he did not bother to look at the list. The surgeon neglected to tell me to stop taking one of those medications, which meant I could not absorb the anesthesia or opiates.

The insult to injury with this situation was that the port was supposed to be so helpful. A port is a small medical appliance, that is installed beneath the skin. A catheter connects the port to a vein. For me, it was used because they could never find a vein when we would do IVs. It was intended to make my treatments more accessible and less painful. While it was the surgeon's error, he blamed the port for never working and always being extremely painful to access.

In a perfect world, this would be an isolated incident. Sadly, I have countless other examples like this one. I also know many different stories from many other people who have had even more traumatic experiences living with chronic illnesses.

Understand me though, and this is not going to be a doctor-bashing book. In my subsequent port surgery, the surgeon was out of this world excellent! Such an exceedingly kind and wonderful human, he promised me that no one in his surgery room would say one negative word about me or my body. He didn't just say it, he meant it. Unfortunately, life with chronic and invisible illnesses is often unpredictable. He had already created the spot for the new port. He took the "defective port" out, although we all know that was the faulty surgeon's error, my body continued to reject the new port. This fantastic human worked for FOUR HOURS to attempt to force my body to comply. My body, however, did not comply and forgot how to play nicely with others, as it often does.

I imagine that if you are reading this book, you either live in a body that frequently does not play nicely or love someone who has a body like that.

Regardless of why you're here, I want to take a few moments and welcome you. I also want to acknowledge that living with chronic illnesses is a huge struggle for many. It is exhausting, disheartening, annoying, and can quickly become all-consuming. Waiting for answers, doing your medical research, not knowing which of the three to five medical providers you should trust, and feeling like your symptoms do not get the time and attention they deserve can all grind you down.

Living with the constant yo-yo recommendations, the darts at a wall diagnosis, the baffling blood work, the bodies that do not work in the way the textbooks explain that they are made or created to work; these are all things that none of us signed up for. Because none of us ever agreed to live in these bodies, I would wager many of us often find it exhausting, frustrating, disheartening, isolating, alienating, defeating, and even dehumanizing. This is not a journey of mere mortals can take, and when the vessel that you are in for this entire journey of life continues to betray you with viruses, bacteria, poor labs, infections, pains, aches, fevers, weight gain, weight loss, etc., it is difficult not to hate the enemy that is your own body. To suggest making peace with your body would be making a mockery of our experiences. I want to suggest something much deeper.

First, however, let us make sure this is for you.

Have you been to multiple providers only to hear the same phrases again and again, like; "but you don't look sick", or "these test results don't make sense", or even "have you tried to exercise or meditation" as if that was some sort of magical cure? How many different providers have you seen where you left with more questions, frustration, rage, hopelessness, or lack of valid answers after repeated appointments? How often do you feel like you are more of an expert on your illness than your medical provider and that you seem to be paying for time to constantly offer education to your medical provider? If you have ever felt so desperate for answers that you would do anything to just put a name or a label on what you are experiencing, then you live in an unwell body. If you have gone to more than one provider for the same issue, yet some are hesitant to get your hopes up about getting real help, odds are you live in a body with an invisible illness. Do you consistently hope that your providers will FINALLY recognize how much you do not feel good, and yet they just keep telling you either that it's getting better, or it will get better? Do you go to the internet looking for information, only to feel minimized because you do not have cancer or some other lethal disease?

To be honest, that list could go on and on, but hopefully, this has given you a glimpse of what I'm referring to. Have you begun to see yourself in the glimpse I've shown you? Let's be honest for a second, if you've stuck it out this far odds are more than likely that you and I have something to talk about. Look, to be honest, I'm not going to include a list of diseases, ailments, and illnesses out of respect and admiration for those people who may have one I may miss; the ones who constantly get overlooked. I want them to know that I see them as much as I see those with cancer. I see every chronic illness person. I see every person pretending to feel good with an invisible illness. I see it because I live it and I understand the ease with which the lie quickly jumps from your mouth to tell even those people you are supposed to "trust", that you are feeling better. Your doctor, your partner, your loved ones, your therapist, your chiropractor all of them get sprayed with the same 'I'm better or fine' lie. It's because you don't dare let someone in that deep. God forbid, you break someone by telling them the ugly truth. The world is probably not ready for that level of destruction.

By the time you finish reading this book, you will be armed with a relentless drive for self-care that gives you actionable steps, rather than just a distracting but ultimately meaningless daydream or fantasy. You will also have a new appreciation for normal in a chronically abnormal body. You will also discover that acceptance isn't the answer to all your problems. The real power lies in the ability to validate. Additionally, you will learn about the freedom and serenity that comes from unapologetically making yourself the number one priority in your own life. I also want you to understand how to set yourself up for success;

to live as much of everyday life as possible for yourself. This book won't protect you from ever getting sick, or having more illnesses pop up. However, I hope that it helps you to develop a heightened awareness of how to be more graceful towards yourself. Which is extremely relevant, when another illness or diagnosis rears its exhausting head, that way you won't have to hide from it. Instead, you can take a deep breath and feel a sense of preparedness.

CHAPTER 2

What Now?

Living with an invisible illness is not only debilitating at times but also downright dehumanizing at others. The very nature of having a disease that other people don't see, recognize, or validate is, in and of itself, disheartening from the beginning. As it continues, it just becomes soul-crushing. I have had so many occurrences of being dismissed due to my weight, my physical illnesses, my energy level, heck, even the hives on my body that at some point, you would think I would become immune to it. Maybe a more accurate description is that my brain can no longer process these experiences, so it just buries them deep.

In all honesty, I had forgotten about the time I went to a Tony Robbins and Pit Bull conference until I was writing this book and my friend reminded me. I just thought I preferred Eminem's music over Pit Bull's. I know I don't have to explain to you all the anticipatory anxiety that occurred before I agreed to go. I inundated my husband with some of the following questions; how we would be flying (because I knew I was too large for one seat. I made him get out the tape measure and see what size the seat was to compare it to my hips), what kind of chairs would we be sitting on at the conference, how far of a walk was it from the parking lot, how much standing was there, they mentioned stairs - did he know how many, what was the walk to the bathroom like? You would have thought he was attempting to get clearance for someone in the President's detail. My husband (who is one of my biggest cheerleaders) worked out all of the tiniest details and soothed even the most neurotic of my anxious questions.

We were going to go and have a great time! We were going to have lunch with Pit Bull. Okay, I'm not going to lie, I had never heard of him before this, but I was still excited. Things seemed okay at first when we got to the event, but I quickly noticed it was mostly an able-bodied event. When the time for lunch with Pit Bull came, I discovered that it was in another building which was quite a walk from where we were. And, unfortunately, it was all uphill. Unlike my wheelchair at home, this rented wheelchair was a manual one. I remember the deep feelings of humiliation and despair. I physically could not walk that far. The pain and exhaustion were just unbearable. And yet my husband just kept pushing me up this steep hill. When we finally got to the lunch, they had all eaten, and we were just shoved at a table. It wasn't the luxurious lunch it had been hyped up to be. Then Pit Bull ran off the stage. I remember thinking, "We paid how much for this!?" The worst part was after the show. Tony's staff was so dismissive of me.

They made me wait until all the higher-paying people had gone so I wouldn't inconvenience anyone. It was mortifying to sit there and watch everyone meets and greet around you and act like you don't exist because you're in a wheelchair.

It's been a while since I've needed to utilize a wheelchair. Even today, though, I still do a mental scan before I commit to something to check if I have the physical energy to see it through. Recently a friend invited me to Disney and I didn't commit because I didn't want to be the one in the wheelchair. At the time, I desperately wanted to walk again without needing a wheelchair, but the more I wanted to not need the wheelchair, the more I needed it. It was as if I was trapped in some freaking reality warp of an alternative world. I would meditate, drink water, not eat carbs, consume no sugar, watch my dairy, and do all of the things the experts said I needed to do, but I just kept finding myself getting sicker and sicker. While I was growing sicker and sicker, I was also feeling increasingly despondent. At the same time, I don't think the irony was lost on me when all the doctors continued to be baffled and just kept giving me the same words, "But you are doing all the right things...." Continuing to do the right things with no reward is a very shallow victory.

I'm going to tell you a tiny little secret. It's not a secret if you know me personally, mostly because I'm not afraid to admit this, and it annoys the ever-loving life out of my husband. Seriously, if we were on a game show and I was asked what annoys him most about me, I would for sure get this one right! I measure the success or failure of medical treatments by making the numbers on the scales decrease. Listen… I never claimed to be the most rational person about all of these things! Honestly, when you have lived in a body that is constantly betraying you while consuming no processed sugar, barely any dairy, and less than 15 carbohydrates a day for over two years, yet the scale keeps climbing like it's on a brisk climb up Mount Everest, you have to focus on something. My specialist continued to tell me that my weight wasn't a result of me overeating or any other factor I have control over. It was simply a result of the toxins in my body, but none of that ever assuaged the devastating humiliation I experienced as the scales topped 388 pounds. I just watched it continue to climb, utterly powerless over the entire experience. Don't get me wrong, and I did all the "right" things. I did South Beach, Atkins, Low-Carb, HCG (even the freaking injections despite my hatred of needles! Ugh needles!), Candida, and Keto! I'm not going to get into the severity and extent of everything I did to drop weight. Let's leave it at the fact that I'm incredibly skilled at being rigid and restricting. If that were a sport, I would qualify for the Olympics. I'd bring home the gold medal, no silver or bronze here, baby!

I have worked with and witnessed enough normal-bodied and healthy humans to see what happens when they have a physical ailment. They schedule an appointment, have the procedure, and BOOM, it's taken care of. To those of us with chronic illnesses trapped in these unwell bodies, that's just literally never been our experience.

Do you know one of my more significant annoyances as a person with several chronic illnesses? It's when everyone and their brother talk about how they chalk it up to brain fog anytime they forget anything. Listen, friends that is NOT brain fog! Brain fog is getting lost when you are just attempting to drive home and you've taken the same dang way home for the last five years. The same way!! Who gets lost like that?! I will tell you who, someone with significant brain fog, and it's no laughing matter, honestly, despite what people say. Also, it's no wonder it's so difficult to live your best life when you're up against those types of issues. I have been accused of being "non-compliant" with my prescribed medications, which is insulting and degrading. If I were in an intimate relationship with these providers, I would flee and never look back. Instead, I continue to pay them and take those heinous accusations. The problem with accusing someone who has a chronic illness, like us, of being non-compliant is that you had better be damned sure that you are accurate before levying such a heavy-weight accusation. We may have brain fog but be sure we will never forget the scorn that sounds like a criminal charge. Come on, it's not like it is willful noncompliance for the sake of disobedience.

As I'm writing this, I received an email from my physician with a change in the supplement regime. I called my husband because my internal response was just, "how am I supposed to remember all of this?!" Even the most foolproof plan is rarely brain fog proof. What's more likely to be the case is it's a case of brain fog causing us to forget what we are supposed to take or when we are supposed to take it.

When the brain fog wins the war, it just hammers down the feelings and emotions to overwhelm us with hopelessness. If feeling overwhelmed and hopeless were raindrops and gumdrops, we'd be in a damn sugar coma!!

I'm not going to sugar-coat this for you because the people who know me and have worked with me would be livid and likely accuse me of hiring a random stranger who had never spent a millisecond with me to write this. Because sugar-coating things, well, that's not my style, honestly. I'm more like blunt honesty wrapped in a whole bunch of grace and love with a heaping dose of accountability type of person. Anything I say will never be in judgment. But let's be honest; will you get the impact if I sugar-coat these messages? NOPE! Me neither!

Let me make this clear; I had my suicide attempt and I laid unconscious on that garage floor (with a double foolproof plan) for three days. I was defeated.

There was no way I could consider doing anything more than existing at that time, let alone being able to live every day as if this was my best life. That was just out of the realm of possibility. While my deepest hope is that none of you ever reach that deep level of desperation, I think most of you can relate to the absolute hopelessness of being unable to find any improvement, of ever getting better. It's challenging to focus on anything positive when you feel a sense of betrayal from your own body.

I like to describe the things that are keeping you stuck as CRAMMED. It's a cute little acronym. It even seems fun, right? When we live with intermittent brain fog, one of the ways we set ourselves up for success is by making things easy for ourselves to remember. Some barriers to living our best life include Confusion, Rabbit holes, Anger, Misdirection, Mistrust, Evasion, and Despair (CRAMMED). Living with the experiences of CRAMMED regularly prevents us from being able to soar with a chronic illness and instead forces us to trudge through one event to the next.

How often are you confused with the massive amounts of confounding or conflicting information out there about your particular illness or disease? Exactly how much time do you spend down various rabbit holes, researching to see if your symptoms match a particular diagnosis, to see what the normal range for lab levels is, to see what milligrams medications and supplements should be taken at? The list is endless.

Then there's anger. This is just a brutal topic, isn't it? There's likely so much untapped anger here for us all. The anger at being ignored, anger at being mistreated, anger about not being listened to, anger about feeling invisible, and anger at oftentimes having more knowledge about your medical complexity than the medical provider you are paying.

Misdirection is so applicable here, isn't it? It often feels intentional, even though logically you know that your providers could not ethically be misdirecting you, right? They wouldn't, they seem like such nice people!

There is so much mistrust when living with a chronic illness. It often feels like a game of darts while blindfolded when you're attempting to ascertain who is trustworthy in your treatment team. The evasion is so deep when you are living with a chronic illness. The medical community will avoid any responsibility or guidance, so you will frequently feel like you are on your own.

The last, but perhaps the deadliest of all these, is the despair. The despair comes in waves and frankly just leaves a tragic mark on you that you can't seem to wash off.

If you have received a formal medical diagnosis for a chronic illness, do you remember those next few days and hours? Did you make any commitments to yourself, vows, promises, or declarations? Where are you now? Where are we all at now?

I remember vividly coming home from my specialist's office and telling my children that I wouldn't be able to keep working as well as cleaning and cooking. They got to choose which I did. The choice they made was for me to keep working so we could keep doing vacations. Duh! They were teenagers. Also, they made some of the most heartwarming promises about dishes and scrubbing floors, the list goes on. I'm here to tell you that they meant every word of what they said at that moment. But they are a lot like typical members of families with chronic illness people. They often seem to have only short-term memory, and their ability to follow through isn't the best. That left me living in a substantial smelly pile of massive guilt! I felt guilt for being sick, shame for being so tired, and responsibility for existing, and I couldn't just sit around and keep asking them for help! Therefore, I did what so many of us living with invisible illnesses do, and really, what those of us with trauma do. Can we be super transparent for a second? If someone tells you that living with a chronic illness isn't traumatic, kick them in the shins. Just kidding, don't do that, but they are misinformed!

Living in an unwell body puts you in a situation where you consistently question your very reality. I can't count how often my friends will message and ask if some physical sensation they are experiencing is "normal" or if they should go to a hospital or seek medical attention. NORMAL people don't wonder if they have a heart attack while cooking dinner for their children. It's not normal for a person to feel their own body and have the sensation of it being on fire, or to have to suffer such an elevated level of pain that most mere mortals would either puke or pass out. Yet, many of us can numb it out and keep moving. This is just a piece of what blocks our ability to live our best life.

When you are constantly sacrificing yourself for the good of everyone else, when you are continually coming in last, when everyone else's needs always have a higher priority than yours, it's going to be difficult to realign your life. Living with a host of invisible illnesses and having your feelings discounted while also questioning your sanity, it's not a difficult leap to understand how those of us with chronic conditions frequently lose our voices. It's also not hard to see why it's such a chore to advocate for ourselves or to fight against so many systems that are not designed to empower us. Let's be honest, most traditional western medicine is not equipped to empower anyone who is not typical, doesn't fit in some definition of 'normal', or is not standard in any way.

Do you recognize the things I have described? Can you see the way you have either surrendered your voice or it has been systemically stolen from you through horrific experience after horrific experiences? Are you beginning to recognize how constantly sacrificing yourself is not serving you, despite working well for those around you because they've been enabled more than a bit? I'm going to ask this one, but it feels pointless; please tell me, if nothing else, if you are exhausted by having to question your very sanity and experiences all the time. Wouldn't it be nice to examine someone else occasionally?! Aren't you just the slightest bit tired of working so diligently to make everything okay for everyone else, and meanwhile feeling so bad on the inside and having to continue to pretend all the time? If you've read this far, then I'm hoping that you are just sick and freaking tired of making everyone else a priority because that is older than that moldy Mac-and-cheese that's in the back right corner of your refrigerator!

If you believe nothing else you read in this book, please acknowledge this utmost truth; you are not alone! Not only are those my experiences, but these are the experiences of my clients and my friends. I also surveyed numerous people I did not know to ensure that I wasn't somehow getting skewed results. I wanted to make sure that my information was accurate, and yes, I'm still a little over the top. What I've talked about, though, are the top issues that prevented people from experiencing the promises I discussed in chapter 1.

My recommendation is to approach this book with as much of an open mind as possible. Listen, I know you've been burned in the past. I also recognize that at this point, you've likely been scammed; you've probably invested several thousand dollars in more than one person who claimed a charming cure that never came to fruition. Then you are left in a huge stinking pile of shame! Hold on, friend; please hold on. I've been there, I have. I'm going to work my butt off not to make any promises I can't keep, and all I ask of you is to keep wading through this book and stay as open-minded as you can. Please know it's okay to set this book down and take your time going through it. Having said that, maybe not the six years it took me to get through the book my therapist recommended I read when I was 19. That changed my life! We all have our paths, right?

CHAPTER 3

Acceptance Is Not The Answer

In typical literary works, most notable authors make glorious promises. I would do the same, promise you the moon and the stars if I knew I could deliver them to you. Let's be very clear for a moment, though. I have lost count of how many times practitioners have made grand promises to me and failed to keep them. I don't want to be just another pretty face to you, though, that might be the first time I've been accused of that. Instead, I would like to make some commitments to you. Would that be acceptable? I commit to you that, by the time you have completed this book, the feeling of isolation and desolation you live with will be lessened. In a perfect world, it would be completely eradicated, but I don't control your internal experiences. You will come to understand that you are not the only one trudging through these experiences. Just keep reading, and together we will uncover so many more truths. I do want to acknowledge that while your brain constantly lies to you and tells you that you are the only one that goes through "X," whatever "X" is, that can't be true.

I'm a clinical social worker by training, and I did some investigative research for this book. One of the findings I came across is that every single year, the percentage of people dealing with long-term health struggles increases. When I went looking a little deeper into the research, I realized there was data that indicated that at minimum 150 million Americans exist with at least one chronic condition. At the same time, around 100 million have more than one chronic condition. And, over 30 million Americans live every day with over five chronic conditions. Tell me again, how this is only happening to you, and you are the only one? I'll wait.

The unique combination of hopelessness, denial, loneliness, confusion, overwhelm, and isolation is brutal. It messes with your mind like no other stressor on the planet. I have a very vivid memory etched in the deepest recesses of my brain from right after I got my initial chronic illness diagnosis. I think it was partially a bit traumatic because I had spent thirty-some years with countless providers in more than four states, all telling me that my problems were just because I was fat, lazy, crazy, and needed to eat less, and exercise more, and the list goes on. It was such a gut punch because, for multiple decades, so many providers had just told me all of my symptoms were "in my head," and my only issue was that I just needed to "lose weight," and now I suddenly found that all that my whole life was a lie. Now I had a label, and it was this?!?! This thing to which there was no cure… This couldn't be true, could it?!?! I would ebb and flow in and out of such a deep state of denial. I remember sitting on my bedroom floor crying, and it was such a deep guttural cry. Do you know the kind? The kind that comes from deep inside your soul? The type you only experience when it feels like someone has reached in and ripped your heart out.

I was sitting on my bedroom floor, the white carpet shaded black because our black puppy's fur spread everywhere. My husband was sitting on the edge of the bed, just looking at me with such complete powerlessness. That's something, I must note, he doesn't experience well, and yet it was a scene we would revisit several times throughout my wellness and healing journey. I remember sobbing and telling him I didn't think I was strong enough to undergo these treatments. Why couldn't he just let me die? I remember the look of pain on his face as he looked at me and explained he didn't know how to live without me, so even if he had to carry me, we were moving forward. So, I, of course, said something trite about him not being strong enough. Then he, of course, said to watch him. In time, I got off the floor, and we plotted our next steps.

So many of us have been taught that acceptance is the answer to all of our problems. I'm here to tell you that's complete and utter garbage. The real secret is validation! When we validate our emotions, frustrations, problems, situations, struggles, and whatever we feel and experience in life, we can find the way through. Remember when that hopeless diagnosis crushed me? Once I validated that, yes, I had been diagnosed with it, the symptoms sucked! The treatment recommendations sucked. Only then was I able to move the huge boulder that had been blocking my path toward a solution. The foundation of everything, for me, always begins with validation. The V isn't for victory for us. It's always for validation!

If you go back to the beginning of this book, you will find some words I wrote in which I made what is best described as a commitment to you. When you finish this book, as they might say in literature, you will take away some conclusions. Because many of you have varying levels of brain fog, I will review them as we go, starting here. I hope you won't find it too redundant. But I also don't want you to have to dig for them. I desire that, when you complete this book, you will be armed with an unabashed drive for self-care that gives you actionable steps rather than just a fantasy and an idealistic daydream. I'm also excited to differentiate between what's normal for you versus what's a problem. So frequently, we spend countless hours attempting to figure out if something should be a concern or a crisis, and we use 'normal' or healthy bodies as our comparison. I've already begun talking about this one. Still, I want you to understand, on a deeper level, that the answer to many struggles is validating your battles, not just blindly accepting them. I am also so excited for you to experience the serenity that will come when you finally shift from prioritizing everyone else to making yourself the number one priority. Lastly, I want to empower you to have a better sense of how to be more grateful towards yourself while living with chronic illnesses. Let's face it, it's a brutal world, and it's even more brutal living in a body that is betraying you.

As we begin to dive into the things that stand in the way of you Soaring with Chronic Illness, and learning how to live every day as if it's your best life, remember not all of these things may apply to you. Please feel free to take what applies to you and leave the rest. While it may not be something that works for you right now, maybe the next time you read this book, it will apply to you. Also, please keep in mind that it's acceptable to 'cut and paste' parts of this. If all of the content doesn't apply to you, but maybe this one section does, feel free to take whatever and however works best for you. My goal is to empower you to live your best life in whatever way is possible with the chronic illness you are dealing with. I'm never going to be able to eradicate your disease because I'm not a scientist, a magician, or a witch. What I can do, however, is help you change how you live with it!

Let me take a moment, then, to give you a preview of what I intend to discuss. These are the tools that have helped me, and I sincerely hope that they can help you too.

C.H.A.R.M.E.D.: Remember the acronym from earlier in this book that you instantly rolled your eyes at? Well, keep those eyes in your head, friend, because this one is going to change your life! Staying focused on living a CHARMED life will allow you to enhance your quality of life and direct the focus of your life away from the pain and suffering.

Living a CHARMED lifestyle almost implies a lavish or luxury lifestyle. What would be different if your life had an air of elegance to it? Please close your eyes for a moment now and imagine it. Can you see it? Can you feel the subtle shifts that happen when you begin to embrace the attitude of a CHARMED lifestyle?

Validation: I have stressed this many times throughout my career and will likely say it until the end of my days. With painful emotions, struggles, turmoil, etc., many of us get caught up and stuck because we want to analyze, evaluate, and judge our feelings and emotional responses. Have you ever had an excited puppy? You know the one, that super obnoxious level of hyper where you often wonder what exactly the dog has been smoking all day. If you've had the experience of an animal like that, then you know that level of acknowledgment where you look at your puppy, and you say something like, "I see you, but I'm not giving you attention right now." That's what I will teach you to do with painful emotions and feelings. It's often described as a game-changer of experience.

No longer being trapped or condemned due to whatever you experience because of your feelings or emotions brings such colossal freedom. More relevantly, imagine having a way not only to cope with but to feel prepared to handle your emotions and feelings. How powerful would that truly feel?

Learning To Advocate for Yourself: The power that this upcoming chapter alone has the potential to provide is immeasurable. It truly is! At this point, I can't even begin to retell the number of stories of medical mismanagement I've heard. Sadly, there are so many stories of patients being mistreated, undertreated, and abused by doctors who should have known better. Doctors who should have done better!

Before hearing other people's stories, I truly believed that I was the only one who'd had experiences like being put through a colonoscopy with no sedation or anxiety medication. Yep, you read that correctly. I was FULLY AWAKE for that one. I'll give you a moment to recover. Here's the thing, though, these kinds of things don't just happen to me. Recently my friend with type 1 diabetes was told she needed to give enough blood for three vials. NOPE! They took blood over SEVERAL hours! And gave her an injection! They also had to keep feeding her during all this! It was a nightmare.

Establishing Healthy and Effective Boundaries: Don't roll your eyes! I get it! Hearing more about boundaries sounds super easy and trite, and like everything else you've read, you probably don't even want to read any further but please at least keep reading this for just a bit longer. When we have healthy and effective boundaries, it helps us stand up for ourselves. It empowers us to have a voice. It gives us the power to say no. It also allows us to shape our preferences, likes, dislikes, wants, and needs. Before providing a voice to our boundaries, we feel that our time, attention, and energy goes to the highest bidder or the one who can play the heaviest emotional card.

The way many of us with chronic illnesses work is that we frequently pay the most attention to those people, situations, issues, and things that are the most demanding or the loudest. The problem with living this way is it's not only exhausting but also challenging to navigate where to focus your attention and energy.

Learning to Embrace your Normalcy: Knowing your own normal is such a crucial yet delicate concept to embrace. It's essential to identify what your standard is, because, without that, you have no baseline. It's like the thermostat in your house. Would you walk in one day and set it to the temperature setting QZ? That would not be very sensible! QZ has no logical meaning for a thermostat. The temperature of 72 degrees, on the other hand, has an agreed-upon or understood meaning.

Learning to embrace your sense of normalcy is about identifying what your highs and lows are, what your danger zones are, what are areas of concern, how to know when it's time to ask for help, as well as knowing when you can navigate things on your own. Without knowing your normalcy, you can't determine any of those.

Set yourself up for success daily: Things have changed for me. I've gone from using a wheelchair to get into my office and having to take naps between my clients to owning a group practice and not even needing a wheelchair when we were on our last two vacations. I can't tell you how huge of a change those were for me! Before you jump on some hugely mistaken soapbox of how I'm different or unique, let me put any ill-founded accusation aside. Trust me! There's nothing special or spectacular about me.

That is unless you count the fact that I have mastered the art of knowing how to set myself up for success like it's a finely tuned, unique art! Success for me has included how to clean my house, get laundry done, write blogs, cook food, enhance my connections with others, etc. Those things are my jam, and I am excited to teach you how to do that as well.

You Alone Determine Your Worth: I long to create a world where we no longer allow our illnesses, diseases, diagnoses, labels, symptoms, or even the lack of any of the previously mentioned to determine our self-worth! What would change in your world if YOU got to choose your self-worth? Not some arbitrary, external, punitively imposed system that seems to be based on keeping you down, but you? Take a few minutes and take an inventory of your health and seemingly "well" friends. Do they struggle with self-esteem and self-worth issues?

The odds are they likely struggle with esteem and worthiness issues on a lesser scale because they are not constantly attempting to compensate for the illness that no one sees. When you are living with a disease that no one else can see, it's not as if you are competing against yourself the way 'normal' people are. No, when you live with chronic illnesses, you are often competing, attempting to garner a shred of self-worth against a host of chronic diseases AND all of the world! How can you be expected to measure up? Stick with me; I have ways.

It's easy to get caught up in the treatment ups and downs, the setbacks and failures, the mounting symptoms, as well as the momentary reprieve in symptoms. All of this quickly mounts to hopelessness, and when coupled with the dehumanizing experiences of being devalued and discounted by countless medical providers, the odds are not in our favor. When we live that rollercoaster lifestyle, is it any wonder many of us lose hope and experience a depressed state?

Please read these words very slowly and very carefully. Being diagnosed with a chronic illness (let alone more than one) is a traumatic experience. We are continually treated unkindly, blamed for our illness if not our symptoms and our statements of compliance with recommendations are discounted. We are often subjected to inhumane medical treatments that would generate a massive outcry if a normal or healthy medical patient were subject to them! Yet we are expected to roll over and give the next vein, cheek, arm, whatever or wherever the injury happened. They want us to take more silently because they don't anticipate us having a voice. I'm here to not only give you your voice back but your quality of life as well. Having an illness is not a moral failing!

CHAPTER 4
C.H.A.R.M.E.D

Courage. Honor. Acknowledgment. Respite. Mastery. Enthusiastic. Dedication

According to a study done by Cleveland Clinic, approximately one-third of all people diagnosed with a chronic illness or disease will experience or exhibit symptoms of depression. That seems like a morbid statistic, Jenn, what's your point? Here's my point; these are just the people who either self-reported symptoms of depression or those whose providers or specialists did the same. Is that okay? Look, can we get honest about something for a second? You and I both know that we are the world's top experts at faking being well. There is no way you can convince me that this number is not a lot higher than that! Therefore, if having a chronic illness creates depression, I want to arm you with something to battle that, so I made the CHARMED mentality.

I'm not going to lie to you. I hope by now, you know that's not my style. There have been times in my life, as a direct result of my chronic illnesses and diseases, that I have been ready to end it all. I have also had the honor to talk my friends and loved ones down off that same wall when their chronic illnesses and diseases became too much to bear. It's a huge cross to bear when you lose the hope of ever getting better. That, coupled with having a brain that is constantly telling you that no one understands and that you are the only one who has ever gone through this, honestly can feel just too much at times. I would do almost anything to prevent you from getting that close to the line.

Have you ever completely and utterly lost hope in your ability to get better? Do you remember hitting emotional rock bottom with your disease? Do you remember the sensation of not having the wherewithal to be able to go to another doctor's appointment? Do you remember that time when you didn't think you could sit in another provider's office and listen to them spew things at you that you didn't believe anymore? Remember that time you just wanted to give up and stop all treatment? I want to explain how staying focused on CHARMED can help with that. It won't eliminate those experiences because it's not a magic wand. It also doesn't give us power over other people, because if it did, well, I wouldn't be here writing this book right now. What it does is provide us with something to stay focused on. It's a mantra or totem to keep our minds on.

Courage: Before you skip right over this one and hurl something trite at me about you, how you don't have any courage, let me stop you right there. You wouldn't be alive right now if you didn't have courage! The human beings I know are actual and exist with the diseases and illnesses we have. That is courage, friends! WE are some of the most courageous people I have ever had the honor of interacting with. It takes a ton of courage for us to wake up every day and face the world again and again. Do not diminish that. If you stopped and focused on how often you had active courage throughout your day, I wonder how surprised you might be by how often you experience it.

Honor: This will be a recurring theme throughout this book. I genuinely hope you will embrace it with every fiber of your being and implement it throughout your life. When my clients begin to honor their bodies, their needs, their desires, their wants, their preferences, their wishes and listen to what THEY need and want, everything begins to shift for them. I want you to find ways to honor yourself. For me, one of the first ways I began celebrating myself was by telling people I was no longer eating foods with nightshades in them Nightshades, no matter how long you cooked them. For those of you not blessed with this devastating allergy, Nightshades include Tomatoes, Potatoes, Eggplant, Peppers, Red Spices (Curry, Chili Pepper, Cayenne Powder, Red Pepper), Paprika, Pimentos, Tobacco, Goji Berries, and Ashwagandha. The massive amounts of hives I got from eating these just weren't worth it afterward, regardless of how delicious it was. Start small and build your ability and willingness to honor yourself. As you become more confident and comfortable, your ability to honor yourself will grow.

Acknowledgment: This is such a pivotal change in perspective to take, so feel free to take notes. Those of us with chronic pain often deny and minimize our pain as a coping mechanism. We have survived in with the "if I don't acknowledge it, then it doesn't exist" mentality. That, my dear friends, is quite frankly, complete, and utter garbage! I do know what I'm about to suggest feels terrifying and is a fundamental paradigm shift, however when you acknowledge your symptoms, your emotions, your feelings, your physical manifestations, and the plethora of other struggles that come with living with chronic diseases, everything begins to shift. Does it eliminate your symptoms? NOPE! Does it magically erase the struggles? NOPE! What it does do, however, is to help to alleviate the mind chatter of "is this real?", "what if someone else isn't experiencing this?", blah blah blah. I'm here to tell you none of that matters. Just acknowledge what you are experiencing and move on.

Respite: This is likely to be a bit controversial. However, based on all of the clients I've worked with who have chronic illnesses, I'm going to unabashedly tell you to REST WHEN YOU CAN! Many human beings are living with chronic pain, chronic illness, and chronic disease. Most people with chronic diseases live with so much shame and guilt that they can't allow themselves to rest outside of predetermined and arbitrary rest times. This just sets you up for more problems. Permit yourself to sleep when you can, prioritize resting, and carve out the appropriate time your body needs to get some true and deep healing. Stop resisting your body's natural desire to heal because some able-bodied human assigned you an arbitrary resting period based on their needs.

Mastery: I like the definition of this word. It fuels my soul when that hopelessness has reached the overwhelming height that makes me feel unable to keep moving forward. One definition of mastery that sticks out for me is; "comprehensive knowledge or skill in a subject or accomplishment." Is that not what each one of us has had to do out of sheer and utter necessity with our chronic illnesses? We've had to become experts on our diseases. We have no one else to rely on; therefore, we must research treatment modalities, coexisting infections, comorbidities, experimental treatment modalities, cross treatment possibilities, etc. We are forced to gain our comprehensive knowledge or skill in chronic diseases! Focus on your mastery skills, and don't allow anyone to cause you to doubt them!

Enthusiastic: Okay, let's cut the crap. You puked a bit in your mouth each time you read that one, didn't you? Like, at some point, you're just getting ready to print out a picture of me, stick it on the wall, and throw darts at it. I can almost hear the accusations being flung at me: Who do I think I am? Don't I know what it's like to have to live with a chronic illness? Do I have any idea how much it sucks?!

Yes, yes, I do! Here's a prime example, just a glimpse into my life. One time, I wanted to take my teenagers to the aquarium. I hadn't understood how my body responded to different temperatures yet. We were taking the wheelchair, though, so I felt pretty unstoppable. And, yeah, it's fantastic to be quicker than these kids! I mean, I'm pretty confident my son was taller than Godzilla, and my daughter wasn't far behind him. Do you know how fast these people walk??!!

Anyway, we get up there, and that city is like 50 degrees colder, plus, here is a news flash - aquariums are freaking cold! My body cramps in painful rolling waves when it gets cold. It's super fun. I couldn't focus on the damn fish in their glass tanks at all. So, yes, I get pained, and I get that life sucks sometimes! But, when you show intense interest in what you are motivated about, things shift for you. Pick your battles, choose where you put your energy. Make sure that you do one thing that you enjoy every single day, even if it's something small.

Dedication: Again, the definition of dedication seems super relevant here; a feeling of very strong support for or loyalty to someone or something. Why will this help you change your quality of life while soaring with a chronic disease? This is such an easy one to answer. You are not an island. While I like to pretend like I'm a modern woman who's badass and independent, I literally could not exist without my support system. Let me tell you a bit about them. My husband is my most prominent advocate, medically speaking. As an ex-EMT, he speaks that medical jargon. Because of my medical trauma history and my propensity to dissociate during medical appointments, he usually goes with me to most of them. Before him, I couldn't even advocate for myself, medically speaking. He's taught me so much in that realm. Then there's my friend, Danielle. She's that friend to whom I can send a picture of any body part, and she will know someone who's experienced it and normalize the heck out of it for me. She's the first one I sent a picture of my black fingers to, by the way. There's my friend Tina who will always offer to help and will sit right beside me during every pedicure, no matter how painful they may seem. I'm sure that sounds silly, how can a pedicure be painful? Trust me, you haven't experienced a pedicure with me! She always has the knack of knowing exactly when I'm at my breaking point and need to have a girl's retreat. There's Jessica, who I have no secrets from. We talk about everything from food, pooping, medical complications, and the list goes on. She's the kind of friend who will point out when my body is misbehaving and express her concern for me and how I'm coping. As I'm crying at home, via text she will help me find clothes in a bigger size. As well, there's Tracy, who is constantly texting me to encourage me to finish this book. While she says it's not a race, she knows everything is a competition to me. Tracy also encourages me to show up in the world and keeps reminding me that I'm worthy of rest. Find, create, establish, and maybe even invite a support system dedicated to you.

I'm going to share a crucial tip with you. Like everything else I teach you, this isn't black and white. You should know, that it's rarely all or nothing when working with me. My best recommendation is to spend a few moments every morning and conceptualize how you would like to implement these things into your life. Close your eyes and take a really deep breath. Where does that feeling of courage exist in your body? Breathe some life into it and see if you can make it grow just a wee bit; even a smidge of growth is better than no movement. Then do that with each of those states; honor, acknowledgment, respite, mastery, enthusiasm, dedication. Pay attention to what shifts and what changes.

Another technique many of my clients respond well to is accountability. Find someone from your support system (out of that dedication realm) and do some accountability check-in with each of these categories. If that makes you feel too vulnerable right now, log it on your cell phone in a habit tracking app, or print out a habit tracker paper and put these words in as the habits you want to track. Find a method that works for you, embrace it, and move forward.

I'm sure I wrote that in a way that sounded super simplistic. Don't get me wrong; I'm not that naive. I know it's not easy. However, if we can make it manageable and simplistic, then it can be achievable. Suppose we make it super complex, then we are all going to get super overwhelmed and ditch it all in a moment of brain fog, pain, or complicated illness. My overall goal is always to set you up for success. Now and always, that is my goal, to set you up for success.

CHAPTER 5

Validation

I'm not going to beat around the bush with you here; I've been sobered since 1996. The foundation of my sobriety was laid with the help of some great and trustworthy friends of Bill Wilson. They will always have a very special place in the innermost recess of my heart. However, both friends of Bill W and pop psychology in general, got a crucial piece of information wrong, as regards a person living successfully with multiple chronic illnesses. Acceptance is very much NOT the answer to all of my problems today! The act of acceptance is often described as embracing the experience, particularly distressing experiences. Is that really what you want to do with your chronic disease? Do you desire to embrace the experience? Hell no! I will go out kicking, fighting, and swinging, but I will not let my disease win and I will not allow anyone else to shame, guilt, or manipulate me into believing that I should! In this chapter, I'm going to teach you how to use validation as a key instrument in your arsenal of tools!

Validation, in and of itself, is the recognition or affirmation that a person, or their feelings or opinions, are valid or worthwhile. If it's a painful, challenging, difficult, (or what some would label 'negative') emotion, feeling, sensation, or state, my biggest and best recommendation to you is to validate that experience. Why? Because by not validating that experience it will simply continue to grow until it becomes unmanageable. It could lead to, for example, an abominable anxiety beast that won't back down from anything. I have just such an experience to share with you. Buckle up, because this is going to be a bumpy story. Are you ready?

When I was informed that all of the fillings needed to be removed from my mouth and that they needed to be taken out by a holistic dentist, I was on board despite my massive dental anxiety. Remember the abominable anxiety monster? This level of anxiety makes that look like a child's toy! In addition to having to see a dentist, which was massively anxiety-producing for me, I also needed to save up $15,000 for this procedure, and also needed both my husband and me to be able to take a week off from our jobs. Since we are both self-employed that meant no income for both of us. So, in total, I needed to save up more than $20,000 because part of the procedure involved a week's worth of hotel stays. I'm sure it sounds over the top to you, but it's because of the complexity of the whole thing and it was complicated by how sick I was. The problem was, of course, that I couldn't even get the money saved up. No matter how hard I tried, the money would just disappear. One crisis after another would drain my account (and that's an entirely different book). Anyway, when my regular dentist decided to do the procedure and just bypass any of the safety measures that ALL OF MY SPECIALISTS said were necessary, I agreed because he was willing to bill it to my insurance. So, my cost went from like $20,000 to about $40. How could I argue with that?! Could you? I mean, could you??

I met with the dentist and agreed with their haphazard plan, even though everything in my body and soul was screaming that this wasn't safe. I, like many of you, have the innate ability to shove that screaming voice into a tiny little box and set that box on fire. As I plowed my way forward, I explained to the dentist how much anxiety I had about this procedure and how little trust I had in dentists in general. Of course, there are drugs for that. I have since lost count of how many tablets they gave me to quash the anxiety. I remember the awe I experienced when I noticed them just stating that they would magically be able to eliminate the anxiety with these tiny pills. It was as if the pills were magic. I did wonder, briefly, if they had forgotten that I was a therapist with an addiction background. I took them as instructed. One the night before at bedtime, one the morning of as I got to their parking lot.

Even then, things began amping up during the appointment though. I cannot remember how many of those pills they had me take while I was trapped in that chair. At one point, they had me attempt to dissolve one under my tongue. They tried the gas, they tried having me listen to my music in my air pods, and they had attempted just about everything. They stopped communicating with me, so I didn't tell them that I had already been using hypnosis to decrease my dental anxiety. Because they weren't talking to me, they had no idea that while I looked coherent, I'd been blacking out. I also had no idea I'd been blacking out until much later… You know, until details just weren't adding up? Like the shake, I demanded my husband buy me as a reward afterward that I then told my son he could have (because I don't like ice cream). After what felt like two minutes, I annoyedly told my son again that the shake was on the counter, and he looked at me like I had three heads and said he had already finished it. There were a whole series of events where I was losing time and I wasn't tracking that I was losing time. I just remember it was like losing my grip on reality but not knowing or not caring, or both, and everything was in slow motion.

When I went through the experience with my specialist, I remember him looking at me as if I was the stupidest person on the planet. One of the things he said to me was, "That was very reckless. If your body had absorbed any of that you could have died." My instant mental response to that? "Huh? Is that why my anxiety was so high? I guess that makes sense then!"

That's exactly why learning the delicate art of validation is so crucial. It looks like sitting down for a cup of coffee with yourself, having a conversation about what's going on, hashing it out, and acknowledging the realness of what's happening. Then it's possible to make an informed decision based on what's happening. Validation is recognizing that you are having an experience, allowing it to occur without getting sent into a tailspin, and moving forward regardless of what that thing is.

For example, I literally can NOT see in the dark. I am blind. Therefore, I stop dead when the lights go out. My husband, however, can see like a cat in the dark. It has annoyed me for the past decade! Every single night, as we shut off the lights to go to bed, I could have a complete come-apart and lose my mind because I don't feel safe in the dark; who knows what's lurking, negative experiences, on and on the list goes. I can't see anything, blah, blah, blah. Instead, though, as the lights go out, I just validate my experience with the darkness. Internally I recognize that I'm not comfortable with the darkness. I may even say something along the lines of, "Hello darkness my old friend type person who I'm going to have no strong feelings towards" I may even sing a copyrighted song about it! Then I grab my phone and turn on my flashlight.

By validating my experiences, it doesn't mean I'm taking up permanent residence there. It just means I recognize the pain or whatever feeling and emotions are at the core of it, and I'm able to pass through it seamlessly. It's like a rock in the river. That rock isn't fighting against the current all day and all night. No, that rock is laying in the water soaking up the sun, just laying there getting polished! It's going with the wave! It sees the water and just goes with it.

Oftentimes well-intentioned people tell those of us with chronic diseases that we need to move into acceptance. I think part of why they push us to do that so quickly is because they are uncomfortable with our discomfort and pain. I'm here to tell you, once and for all, that whatever you are feeling, it is natural and perfectly permissible! There are no such things as bad, negative, or wrong emotions or feelings. Anyone who believes otherwise clearly just doesn't understand how to process feelings and emotions.

Several therapeutic modalities back up my line of thinking, just so you don't think I'm blowing smoke up your butt. Emotional Focused Therapy, Acceptance and Commitment Therapy, the list goes on. Recognizing your own experiences and internal chatter about those experiences is crucial to the healing process. Whether that's physical healing, emotional healing, spiritual healing, or energetic healing is of no consequence. In my work with clients, and my healing journey, the foundation is always built on validation.

Trust me, I get how I'm making this sound super simplistic and how overwhelming this must feel. Remember when I was sitting on my bedroom floor crying about being gutted due to receiving that diagnosis? My husband and I don't share the same beliefs about responding to feelings and emotions. Now that's fine because we are two separate people. He believes that by validating the "negative" feelings/emotions" a person will inadvertently attract more of those 'negative' situations to themselves. In over 25 years of providing clinical therapy to human beings, I've never witnessed that occur. When I was on that bedroom floor, however, he attempted to motivate me through that process, his way of seeing the situation. His motivation was so vile I could have set his very soul on fire.

I rejected his absurd suggestion and navigated my way through that ebbing and flowing denial process, as messy and raw and real as it was. Trust me, it was every one of those things at times! My best suggestion, if you are not familiar with how validating truly works, is to think about any time you might have been around a rambunctious three-year-old. You know how they just get louder and louder and louder until FINALLY; you acknowledge them. If you are around children regularly, you soon learn how to quickly acknowledge the child lovingly and somewhat quietly and move on. Kind of like an "I see you there" and go back about your life. That's exactly what I want you to begin doing with anything that life, your body, the world, whatever, throws at you. Just validate that you see it even if you can't process it fully at that moment. The key is to focus on the fact that validation helps lessen the pressure cooker that we are always experiencing in life.

If you get stuck or overwhelmed, just take a deep breath and ask yourself what are you experiencing at this moment? That's right here, right now, at this moment. What is coming up for you? Just check in with yourself and notice what is happening to you. All you have to focus on is right here, right now, in this one moment. Take it literally one moment at a time. You got this!

CHAPTER 6

Learning To Advocate for Ourselves

If you are going to do more than just exist with your chronic disease, you must learn how to advocate for yourself. Listen, I get it and I hear your complaints and your arguments. I do. I truly understand how much the medical community has discarded and disregarded you. My closest friends have shown up for a simple blood draw only to learn at that very point the medical professionals were doing an invasive procedure. One of my closest friends, as I'm writing this, is struggling with having been kept on a liquid diet for over a month because her doctor just keeps jacking her around. Oftentimes when we don't have the words or skills to advocate for ourselves (or someone else to advocate on our behalf), it feels as if medical specialists will just run right over us. It often feels like they have no regard for our well-being or welfare.

When we don't have the skills, capacity, willingness, or ability to advocate for ourselves things go wrong. Bad things happen. Things go south in a hurry. It's kind of like the time I saw a bunch of different medical specialists for rectal bleeding and they thought it happened because of a previous sexual assault so they wanted me to do a colonoscopy. You just know that's what every sexual assault survivor wants to do, particularly one with a whole host of chronic diseases and illnesses! Sign me up for that one please and thank you so very much! I also know so many of you reading this are going to want to sign up next right? But wait, it gets so much better! I specifically asked if they could give me something for the anxiety because I was so anxious about the entire procedure, and I had no one there for support. I mean, my ex-husband dropped me off and was going to pick me up afterward but that was about it. Let me draw the scene for you; I'm scared, so very sick, and wide the hell awake through this entire procedure. You see, not only did they refuse to give me anything for anxiety, but they also refused to give me anything for sedation. I vividly remember that I just didn't understand how most 50-year-old men just willingly signed up for this, especially when the scope got stuck inside me and they were just jerking and jerking and jerking trying to get it unstuck. The whole time, I'm just laying there gripping the side of the table as if the earth will eventually fly so fast it'll spin me off. I remember going back to work afterward, and a few of the over 50-year-old men that I worked with at that time were shocked that I was back at work so soon. They each looked at me and said the same thing, "How are you back at work already?" That response confused and baffled me. It would take me years to piece together the information and realize that most people were sedated for something like that.

When we don't have a voice and we don't have a way to ask important medical questions, then we don't assert ourselves and ask the necessary questions. We don't get properly educated. Even just learning how to ask for help is important. We need to be able to say things like; hey I do not understand this, I need help, can you please slow down and explain this to me, I'm not following, these hurt, do better, and the list goes on. All of these phrases are crucial as you develop the skills to advocate for yourself.

I've been seeing a chiropractor since I was an infant. There's a family history about how I had bacterial pneumonia four times before I was a year old and the doctor had told my parents to call the priest for last rites. One of the guys my dad worked with suggested seeing a chiropractor. Forty some years later, I still attribute so much of my functioning to mine! Here's what I love about Dr. Johnson; he listens and talks in ways normal people can understand. When I went in to see him after my specialist blew me off with some medical jargon about a Herxheimer response that I needed to watch out for, it was Dr. Johnson who, when I mentioned it, took the time to slowly and in simple everyday language explain it to me. Not just once either, he kept finding ways to point it out to me when it would show up so I could see what it looked like in my life. He was only able to do that because I explained to him that I had no idea what a Herxheimer response was. Okay, truthfully, I couldn't remember what it was. I had to Facebook message him when I got back home, but you get the point!

Learning how to ask for help, say no, use your voice, ask for what you want or need, and be prepared to get up and walk out of a medical appointment are all the things that will make you your own best advocate. Another thing I will recommend is for you to keep a notebook or a three-ring binder (or both) with you that you bring to medical appointments. At one point, when I was super organized, I kept all my labs, copies of blood work, receipts from medical appointments, summaries from specialists and other medical providers, x-rays, etc. all in one three-ring binder. However, because I don't always find it easy to write in a three-ring binder, I just bring that along to put the documents in. However, I have also previously typed up a list of questions and added them to that three-ring binder. Otherwise, I will just write them in the notebook, making sure to leave enough room to add the answer.

Unless you are going to the emergency room, have a plan for every medical appointment you go to. For the longest time due to an extensive history of medical trauma, I had no voice at all. We would go to see my amazing chiropractor, Dr. Johnson, and he would ask whatever question he normally asks. I literally cannot find that question in my brain as I am sitting here typing right now. It's such a benign question about how you are doing or where the discomfort is, but for YEARS it made me freeze. Therefore, I gave him my canned and stock response, the one I gave to able-bodied people who were not safe and not in the "know". Essentially, he would walk into the adjustment bay and greet me, and I would freeze. Thankfully my husband was there for the longest time to translate. Because I work to advocate for myself and weed through providers to make sure I have high-quality providers; I have a chiropractor who I can trust and who's trauma informed. So, he did the work to unpack what my 'good' or 'fine' meant. These days, I can tell him things like, "I've had a migraine for 7 days" or "this leg has been numb and electrocuting me for two weeks". I know he's not going to mock me, belittle me, humiliate me, question me, or judge me.

I have a similar relationship with my primary care, Dr. Rohde. In all honesty, at this point today, despite years of medical trauma and being blamed for all my medical issues, I feel 100% confident going to see Dr. Rohde alone. Why? Because I've cultivated that relationship. I've laid my neurosis on the table. Does he love that I judge the success or failure of a treatment modality by seeing if I drop weight? Uhm, definitely not! He does poke a bit at that when it comes up and we all laugh about it because I can recognize that it is irrational. Here's why I will continue to see him regardless; he has all of my buy-ins! He has done so much research on the irregularities of my body! He "jokes" about how my body just can't follow the textbook, because it honestly can't. Importantly, when he arrives at the appointment, he's done his homework! He's graphed out his reports, he's mapped out the labs, and he's put the pieces together to show me a story of why things are the way they are.

I have this level of provider because I continue to advocate for myself. When I had a provider who was only willing to test my hormones and other lab work every six months despite me suffering from covid long haulers because they had grown too busy, I stopped going there. Did I feel bad? Absolutely not! I'm paying for a service. Would you continue to go to the same restaurant if every time you went there, they served you burned grilled cheese instead of lightly toasted it? Then why, under some false sense of guilt or shame, do we keep going to someone just because they have a medical license?

Learning how to advocate for yourself begins with standing up for yourself, using your voice, saying no, permitting yourself to take up space, allowing yourself to acknowledge the discomfort and pain and needs that you experience, demanding to be spoken to rather than about, and forcing medical providers to treat you like a human being rather than a number or a statistic. It starts by telling providers when they are hurting you physically or causing you pain. It starts when you tell a provider that they hurt your feelings, have been too harsh, or have just been thoughtless. It begins when you say that they can no longer continue to make idle threats about a worst-case scenario as if you don't exist. It begins when you take a stand (no matter how big it feels or how tiny it looks). It begins when you cancel an appointment with a provider who treated you poorly or talked down to you. In essence, it starts when you choose yourself. Learning how to advocate for yourself will be a daily journey that continues every time you make a decision that shows that you are supporting yourself, that shows you are making decisions that are in your best interest, that demonstrates you are becoming your own best medical advocate.

Here's a quick and dirty how-to if you want to fast-track the learning process here. I'm all about some effective shortcuts. Do you know anyone who is just a super stellar advocate? Do you remember the scene in Designing Women when Julia went to see that doctor who blew off her friend's doctor? I remember how she laid into him for disregarding the missed breast cancer. She did so with such firmness, tact, grace, and yet just a bit of intimidation. I've always wanted to develop that communication style. Instead, my style is more like sass, sarcasm, assertiveness, a wee bit of aggression, and bluntness. If you don't have someone in your life who you can use as a role model, then, go to YouTube and watch that scene. Look for people who are strong role models and good advocates and then mimic their behaviors. When you are engaging with medical professionals who are not treating you the way you need to be treated, embody those people and imitate those behaviors. I'm sure you will be thrilled with the results. It's been a game-changer for me and I trust that with some diligent effort it will be for you as well.

CHAPTER 7

Learning How to Establish Healthy Boundaries

isten, friends, I've been a therapist for over twenty-five years. The facial expression and response when I introduce this concept of healthy boundaries to clients (and friends for that matter) have not changed one single bit. There's typically an element of overwhelm, there's a spot of confusion, there's a strong hint of an outright denial, and then there's straight-up defiance. Frequently, those of us with chronic diseases think we don't need boundaries for some archaic reason. Every living breathing human being needs boundaries! It helps me to know where I begin, and I end. It's like houses, right? A boundary is a line that tells us where the property line is, where my place stops and your place starts. However, our internal resistance makes a lot of sense when you think about it. When you look at dysfunctional family systems and see how many people are raised with covert family rules, including things like, don't talk, don't feel, don't think, and don't trust, then to me, it is no wonder that so many human beings struggle with enacting effective boundaries. I understand that it's scary and feels overwhelming. However, implementing boundaries has allowed my friends to begin to advocate for themselves at their medical appointments. It also allowed me to tell people, thank you so much for passing along what "cured" their fifth cousins, ex-spouses, a neighbor from down the street, and twice removed dead aunt from the same disease I have, but I'm going to trust the providers who have looked at my actual blood work, or who have a medical degree.

Here's where the problem for those of us with chronic illnesses exists when it comes to having or establishing boundaries. Typically, we have such a high level of guilt and shame for being sick, for being a burden on those who love us, for not being able to carry our "share of the weight" (whatever that means), and the list goes on. The struggle is that most of us with a chronic disease are people-pleasers. Whether we were people-pleasers before the diagnosis or symptoms of the illness and disease is irrelevant at this time, because here we are. We all have to get to the point where our boundaries are stronger than our need or desire to please other people.

In the early 1990s, when the Oprah Show was still airing on television, I called my mom and asked her to set the VCR to record an episode (for those of you not in the know, a VCR is basically like a DVR but it's an external machine). I wasn't a regular viewer of the Oprah show but I was super excited and intrigued by this episode because whoever it was that was on the episode (I no longer remember exactly who) was talking about boundaries. Whoever they were, they shared some life-altering information (at least for me) that I continue to share with my clients to this day.

One of the biggest lessons I learned was to not commit to anything at the moment. I learned how to change my default setting to, "I need to check my schedule and get back to you." What responding with this does, is allow us some emotional space to figure out if we have the physical or emotional energy or ability to engage in whatever the requested activity is. It allows us to figure out if we even want to engage in the activity. So often, when living with a chronic disease, we just arbitrarily agree to everything out of guilt and shame rather than checking in with ourselves to see if it's something we have the time and energy for. Or, and here's a shocking concept, do you even want to do it!!??

For the longest time, especially at the beginning of my disease, I would just arbitrarily say yes to anything. This was partly because I was terrified of being left behind, but also because I had such an overabundance of guilt and shame that I was drowning in it. Giving myself that freedom from having to answer immediately was such a huge relief. Every time I answer out of some obligation or presumed pressure and don't give myself that space, I instantly regret it. Then, of course, I am stuck in this huge sucking void of do I cancel, do I not show up, am I honest, can they handle the truth, do I make up something that sounds socially acceptable, do I cancel at the last moment citing some other emergency, how am I supposed to get out of this because I just can't go?

Boundaries are crucial when you have chronic diseases because you are living with impaired energy levels, possibly chronic pain and various other health issues including coordination complications, brain fog, difficulty breathing, vision issues, mobility issues, hearing concerns, digestive issues, and... the list feels like it just does not stop at times. When you are at war with your own body, it's imperative to be able to set limits with people who are offering suggestions for what they believe is best for your body. People are telling you how you can be more productive, telling you to just push through, assuming you "don't look sick", and making wildly inappropriate assumptions based on your body size or function. That's another list that could go on forever.

When I'm working with people to help them learn boundaries, I go back to that Oprah episode. I remember that unknown lady suggesting that there are three sentences to complete. They are:

People may not________________________.

I have a right to ask for________________.

To protect my time and energy, it's okay to________________.

Typically, when I'm working with people to establish boundaries, I suggest they complete these sentences between ten and fifteen times.

Some examples when I'm working with people who have chronic diseases include; people may not offer me "suggestions" without my consent, people may not comment on my body, and people may not criticize my productivity. Other examples include; I have a right to ask for help, I have a right to ask for guidance, I have a right to ask for space, and I have a right to ask for security. The suggestions to fill in the blank in the last sentence include are things like, to protect my time and energy; it's okay to rest, it's okay to change my mind, and it's okay to say no.

The crucial pieces to being able to effectively implement solid boundaries include knowing what you need, being able to recognize your limits, prioritizing your healing, and recognizing that you are going to have to find a way to advocate for yourself (Is this Deja vu or is there a chapter about that?).

Here's something you need to be aware of, that may be uncomfortable, as you move forward in your journey to survive your chronic disease; you will lose some relationships as you attempt to recover from your chronic disease. One of your boundaries need to be to prioritize your healing, so you will need to learn to develop a shield of armor so people's opinions and beliefs don't crush your soul or have as strong of an impact as they used to. Above all else always remember that you deserve to heal! No matter how bad it feels when someone rejects you because you are sick or because you can't go to dinner anymore (or book club, or yoga, or whatever the thing is!) please keep your eyes on the prize.

WE are always the prize, friends. I don't care who thinks that's arrogant. I will apologize to no one for it! I hope that you can get to the point where you can recognize the power that knowing, seeing, and envisioning your boundaries bring you. I know that when you begin to entertain boundaries it feels like sheer arrogance. In reality, however, it's confidence. It's a necessary amount of self-efficacy. It's the essential element of survival.

Once you get skilled at it, you will find yourself asserting boundaries all over the place. I recently left a provider who is very pleasant and honestly a great human being with a delightful heart. The front desk staff, on the other hand, are abhorrent, and they've grown too big that they no longer provide the level of care I prefer. I had Covid pneumonia and less than four months later they arbitrarily changed their entire system. Now instead of doing my entire hormone blood work every three months (which, given how wonky my body is, I believe is necessary), they refuse to do it any more often than every six months. Well, that just didn't work for me, honestly! I was on the cusp of dealing with a crap ton of post-Covid stuff and not loving the impact it was having. Do you know what I did? I took my business to a place where they respect me and communicate with me about the frequency of my appointments and lab tests. It's delightful. In a shocking turn of events, science and testing here are so much more effective! Who knew?

An example of what boundaries look like for me in terms of personal relationships is that I'm no longer available for one-sided relationships. That's just a hard no for me. I hope it already is for you and me telling you this is just redundant. If not, though, keep reading. As a business owner, Covid was a terrifying time. We all had to work from home. Because of the complexity of my illnesses, the only time I left the house for four months was to go on walks. At the same time, I had this entire business to keep open. I committed text my friends who were business owners every single day, to check in on them, see how they were doing, see if they needed anything, how they were holding up, you know - the whole works. The friends who are real friends also developed that same habit and it kind of became a game, who could text whom first. There were some people, though, who just sucked me dry. They just took all of the attention and empathy and compassion I would dish out until I realized it was so one-sided. There were those few 'friends' who never inquired about how we were doing, how we are holding up, how the move went, did we need anything, did we need any extra assistance while dealing with Covid pneumonia? I'm prepared to admit I'm always a slow learner with these things, but when I learn it and reach that point, I will end things fairly abruptly. There's no such thing for me as being undone. When people are that selfish and self-centered, we don't need that level of time and energy being sucked out of us.

Boundaries are another way of, honestly, just choosing you! Living with a chronic disease and illness will warp your self-esteem and self-confidence if you don't hedge against it. I want our boundaries to be rock solid so that regardless of how our diseases manifest, regardless of what that does to us, or what it looks like, we can recognize the amazing human beings we are and how much worth we bring to the table.

Speaking of tables, can we stop inviting people to sit at our table who don't deserve a seat there anymore? Can you stop inviting people to sit at our table who are going to put us down for honoring our bodies and focusing on our healing? Can we please stop setting a place at our tables for people who are going to talk trash about our need to prioritize our healing?!

If you are not on board with what my healing looks like or needs to include, find a different table. Healing is such a high priority in my life!

CHAPTER 8

Learning to Embrace your Normalcy:

The definition of normalcy is; the condition of being normal the state of being usual, typical, or expected. When you conceptualize living with chronic illness, chronic pain, or chronic disease the mere concept of normalcy almost seems like an oxymoron doesn't it? However, think about the Covid pandemic for a moment. How many times do you remember hearing people talking about how we just needed to get back to "normal"? Everyone is always working toward or attempting to establish normal, no matter what it means or feels like for them. What I want you to understand is that my normal is different from your normal, which is different from his normal, which is different from her normal. Which is a long-winded way of saying every single living human being's sense of normalcy is different.

Something many people just gloss over is the maddening feeling of betrayal and absolute rage that you are likely to experience at times when living with a disease, pain, or illness that causes you to feel as if you are at war with your own body. The amount of gut wrenching rage many chronic diseases sufferers experience because we can't make sense of our bodies is almost beyond understanding. I spent vast amounts of time and energy trying to make everything make sense in my brain. I saw energy workers, hypnotherapists, therapists, bodyworkers, acupuncturists, mind-body specialists, naturopaths, etc. If there was a specialist out there, I saw them. I worked my butt off because people kept acting as if my mindset somehow would magically cure my physical health. Listen, people, I spent hours each day guarding my thoughts, meditating, doing self-hypnosis, journaling, and so on. I was doing all of these things! I mentioned previously that I can do things to the extreme, right? Well, this is merely another example!

When people are dumping toxic guilt and shame on you, and you haven't carved out the space yet to grieve for the loss of a healthy body, you can struggle with what normal is for your own body. I've been present and held space for so many people who have struggled with knowing if something was normal while using someone else as an arbitrary measuring stick.

My friend, Sally, went to the ER because she was experiencing massive pain and a 'slight' fever. The emergency room decided that she was not really in pain so they did no real blood work or scans and sent her home. Because Sally had no baseline for what was normal for her and no ability to advocate for herself, she just went home as instructed because, after all, they were the "doctors". Turns out, that Sally actually had a ruptured appendix and became septic. It was really brutal and touch and go for her for a while. What happened to Sally happens to people every single day, especially those of us with chronic diseases. We are often tossed aside, our symptoms minimized, our experiences discounted, and we are left to fend for ourselves.

Another example of something similar occurred to my good friend Steve. Steve kept having intermittent stabbing pain in his shoulder. He kept bringing it up with his primary care physician, but his PCP kept telling him it seemed fine to him (based on no x-rays, ultrasounds, MRIs, or any other tests). Over time, Steve ended up in the emergency room numerous times. The problem is, when you have chronic diseases or chronic pain, they traditionally act as if you are just a cry baby or a drug seeker. Anyway, they kept blowing Steve off until finally, some doctor discovered he had blown at least one disc in his neck. I don't remember how many, but I do remember the doctor being confused about his continued ability to function.

I want to empower you to not measure what's normal for you compared to what's normal for me - or Joe Smith, or Steve Jones, or my dog, or anyone else on the planet. I want you to have the inner fortitude and conviction to just know that, "hey THIS doesn't feel right (or isn't right) so I want it addressed, now please". I want to give you some mantras that may help you to stay focused on learning to embrace your normalcy. They include:

I know I am worthy of meeting my own needs

I can give a voice to my discomfort

I know my own needs

I am in touch with my sense of normal.

I know I am fine-tuning using my voice.

Mantras or affirmations are powerful ways to program your subconscious mind. You can write them, sign them, say them, speak them, chant them, doodle them, draw them, color them, or even imagine or visualize them coming true every night as you go to sleep. Part of the challenge is that many of us have so much subconscious mental programming that tells us we must not make a fuss. Your mind may have these ideas. Don't make a scene. Don't be a bother. Don't be a nuisance. Don't create any extra work for people, because we all know damn well that the mere existence of our chronic disease is already creating so much extra work for the entire world. We ought to just issue apologies to people that pass us on the street.

Imagine for a moment, just humor me for a second, okay, because what I'm about to say is going to sound bizarre. However, imagine that your opinion is valid right here, right now. It's valid without any confirmation, without any outside opinions, without sending pictures, without calling five people and confirming, without fact-checking your symptoms on Google, without doing whatever else you need to do to convince yourself that it's acceptable to reach out and get medical treatment.

How different would it be to just simply trust your own opinion? Have you had that experience where someone attempted to convince you of something that you just inherently believed was wrong? You know the situation, no matter what they said your opinion could not be swayed because you just knew that you knew whatever it was. Unless they presented you with cold hard scientific data you were certain not to change your mind, and even then, the evidence would have to be pretty amazing to make you reconsider at all. That's the level of unquestioning, unwavering confidence I want you to have in your sense of normalcy!

Resign from the debate committee, stop analyzing every symptom and every ache and pain, and trust yourself! Get quiet and listen to that voice inside of you, the one that tells you when there's an issue or a problem. My friend Danielle recently had an experience where she wasn't listening to that voice, and what she kept dismissing as a sore throat ended up being a horrible case of pneumonia.

Let me ask you a question, have you ever been around a young child? Specifically, have you been around a child around three or four years old? They are my favorite ages on the planet, honestly! That's because they have an unfiltered and unwavering belief in every single thing you say, right? What if you begin treating yourself like that three- or four-year-old? This is one of the most powerful ways to empower your sense of normalcy. Treat your desire to establish a sense of normalcy like your interactions with a small child. Get curious about it. Be positive towards it.

Another aspect of normalcy that you need to consider when living with a chronic disease is establishing your level of external normalcy. When your body is creating havoc and putting you through war, it's crucial to your survival for you to create a solid foundation of normalcy in your daily life. What that looks like is establishing routines around yourself as much as you can. Routines and rituals are such healing activities for most people. There's a significant amount of research that points to how healing rituals are for our brains. Many of us think of rituals from a holiday, birthday, or anniversary perspective. However, take a few moments and explore your everyday rituals. What are your cooking rituals, what are your eating rituals, what are your rituals around paying bills, and what are your rituals around connection?

Let me explain some rituals from my life for a little bit. Every Wednesday at 1 pm I go to lunch with Jessica, because she helps me to stay grounded. We work together and our offices are right next to each other but leaving the building and going out for lunch creates a whole other level of ritual. Another ritual of connection I have is that once a month I go with my friend, Tina to get a pedicure. It's not about the pedicures at all. It's about pampering and having downtime to connect. A ritual around food I have is that one day over the weekend, I typically spend a few hours preparing meals for the week and freeze at least a portion of the food. Yes, the holiday, birthday, and anniversary rituals are important to me as well. It is these daily rituals, however, that sustain me through life and help establish my sense of normalcy.

The final aspect that's important to consider when looking at your sense of normalcy is to manage your expectations. When you begin medication or a treatment regime, it's important to remain hopeful that you can get better while also being mindful of just how much hope and faith you put into this pathway. No matter what happens, don't let it get you down. Remain steadfast in moving forward and remain committed to the concept that you are never giving up.

It's also crucial to managing your expectations of other people. People aren't superhuman, therefore they are going to screw up. The average person, unless they have a chronic disease, is rarely going to be compassionate toward what we are going through. At one point or another, they will also likely make promises they don't keep, they will say things they don't inherently mean, and they will fail to keep commitments at various points. I always say that people are so human! If only they were dogs, how much better the world would be. I'm a huge proponent of managing and checking our expectations. Whenever I'm disturbed or upset, my goal is to check my expectations. To be clear, I'm not telling you to have any expectations because that leads you to a whole set of other issues. When we set our expectations too low it leads to people walking all over us. The optimal place to be with expectations is in the middle of the road. We never want our expectations to be too high (because that always leads to instant disappointment) or too low (because that leads to us being devastated).

Remember that you, alone, establish your sense of normalcy. While the biggest sense of normalcy that many of us struggle with is the internal normalcy in our bodies, it is paramount to establish a sense of normalcy outside of our bodies in our daily lives as well.

CHAPTER 9

Set Yourself Up for Success Daily:

This is perhaps the most important concept. It's one that helped me reconsider the idea that I was going to have to stop working and serving my clients, which feeds my soul and just stay at home every day. If I consider myself an expert at anything, it's setting myself up for success. I understand many of you are exhausted, burned out, and overwhelmed. Honestly, I'm a huge proponent of conserving our energy when we can. Learning how to set ourselves up for success is a complete paradigm shift for so many of us who have spent our lives engaged in apologetic lifestyles where we seem to have to atone for our mere existence let alone for the heaping pile of chronic diseases on top of it! The first step in setting yourself up for success daily is to stop apologizing for your disease, stop apologizing for being in pain, stop apologizing for your illness, etc. It's not a crime to need accommodations, and let's ask ourselves how often we make allowances for everyone else in our life. Setting myself up for success daily is one of my biggest superweapons, honestly. I've become an absolute rock star at constantly navigating ways to adapt my situation to make it work for me. Honestly, it's such an intuitive part of who I am and what I do now, that most people don't even know that I'm doing it.

When I worked by myself (before owning a group practice), and used a wheelchair to get to the office and in public, I would strategically schedule my clients in such a way that I could take a two-hour nap without interfering with my ability to see them and provide good care. It wouldn't negatively impact my ability to make a livable wage either. That's just me, things I've helped my friends and clients implement to set themselves up for success daily include; setting reminder alarms on their cell phones with the name of the medication or supplement they need to take at a specific time, coming up with a color-coded medication container system, outsourcing their laundry because their pain or energy does not allow them to engage in doing it on their own, getting a housekeeper to help with the deep cleaning or offset the chemical smells that trigger so many people with chronic diseases or chronic pain issues, or even how to manage your time with chronic diseases.

Jeannie was in danger of losing her job because she was just consistently late for work. Her employer directed her to have NUMEROUS conversations with Human Resources. Despite their best intentions and greatest suggestions, however, HR just couldn't help Jeannie get to work on time. Jeannie's employer also made several recommendations/ orders for Jeannie to engage in traditional talk therapy. The problem was that none of these therapists were skilled or knowledgeable in working with chronic illness, chronic pain, or chronic disease. Once I began teaching Jeannie how time management is different for those of us with chronic diseases, she began setting herself up for success daily and wasn't late for work again except in the case of an unforeseen emergency. That was an absolute game-changer for her!

The first specific way that I homed in on setting myself up for success daily was understanding that time and time management just work differently for me. I work diligently to put no judgment and no value on that concept because I'm also reconciled to the fact, I can't change that. Trust me, I diligently worked to change it, and it wouldn't budge. Therefore, when it crops up as an annoyance, I just validate that annoyance or frustration and focus on how I'm going to address it. The reality is when your physical, cognitive, emotional, and relational energy is frequently wonky it's crucial to find a system that works for you. It's important to come to terms with the fact that it's going to look different from day to day and from moment to moment. My time management skills when I have minimal brain fog are hugely different compared to my time management skills when my brain fog is so heavy, that I can't locate my address in my brain, or when I can't find my way home without using GPS. While I don't plan for crises, I do have backup contingency plans because then I don't have the stress and anxiety of worrying about whether or not something goes wrong.

My default answer is always the same these days, I just pull out the backup plan.

If you are a person who tends to measure your self-worth based on your productivity it becomes difficult to navigate a chronic disease. Oftentimes this amplifies the negative self-talk that coexists with an invisible illness. If this, is you, I recommend doing a lot of the prep work the night before. This includes having your keys, lunch, work bag, clothes, and shoes set out the previous evening. There was a point in time where every night before I went to bed, everything was laid out for the next day. Mornings were such a struggle for me as I didn't sleep well and that, in combination with my oxygen dropping so low during the night, made things difficult. Mornings felt like trudging through wet cement with sandbags on my feet. I was unwilling to give up because I had bills to pay and, honestly, my pride just wouldn't allow it.

I still fall back on the night before philosophy when I'm facing a serious level of exhaustion, when my brain fog is super high, when my pain is extraordinary, etc. One of the things I like about engaging in that process is it sets my mornings up to be smoother, more organized, less complicated, and honestly just so much easier overall. In a perfect world, I would be one of those people who'd have five or seven days' worth of outfits set out at a time. Do you know what that looks like? The whole outfit from the panties to the socks! The whole outfit from head to foot. So, I could just walk in there, grab an outfit, and go. That just sounds so pleasing to me. However, my brain doesn't organize things quite that well. Therefore, I compromise in other ways. For example, all my shirts and dresses get hung in the closet. My jeans go in the dresser drawer, and my leggings go in the drawer in the closet. Guess what? What happens if I don't find the energy to put the clothes away that week? Nobody dies and nobody goes to jail! Everyone is safe and has a place to sleep. Therefore, it's not a crisis or an emergency.

Another quick and easy way that I set myself up for success is to prepare food in advance. Food prepping is something that decreases my overall stress, as it does for many people. Part of why it is overall a relaxing activity is because it stimulates the parasympathetic nervous system, which creates the sensation of being calm, relaxed, and grounded. Any time you do anything creative it stimulates the parasympathetic nervous system. When the system begins to activate, as you start the creative activity, it may feel like tiredness to you because you are not used to the relaxed state. At any rate, I used to cook a couple of big meals on Saturday and Sunday and eat the leftovers throughout the week as well as share them with my family. We'd use them for lunches and dinners. However, what happened for me is those leftovers began creating histamine responses and were very unsafe for me to eat. Again, I had to get creative. Currently, my approach is to cook a big meal on my days off and freeze those leftovers. Here's the compromise I've made with myself though. As I'm preparing to freeze it, I will put a bigger container in the refrigerator for my family who can then eat leftovers all week. I put individual servings in the freezer for myself. Then I just take them out, cook them, and eat them. So far, I've not had a histamine reaction. The key to setting yourself up for success is to remember that nothing can defeat you unless you allow it to, and it's crucial to remain flexible when living with a chronic disease that can throw another pile of yuck at you!

A further important strategy in setting myself up for success is learning how to implement batching to conserve energy. My experience of introducing batching into my life was an absolute game-changer in managing my chronic disease. Batching is typically defined as grouping tasks together in a way that you can do them all at once, rather than jumping back and forth between tasks that take place in different programs or areas. This was a key element in conserving energy, decreasing pain, and maintaining my mental health during the height of my illnesses. Whenever I have a flare-up of symptoms, it's what I always go back to. However, here's my warning; people will often mistake batching for laziness. Even my husband, who is probably one of my biggest supporters, often misunderstands my batching attempts for laziness or lack of effort. For me batching is not carrying the laundry to the laundry room until you have a full load, it's not running to the bank until you have a deposit that justifies the time and energy that it will involve, its food prepping a few meals at a time instead of just one or two (to conserve the energy and pain it may involve), stacking up all the errands instead of doing errands every day, etc. It's conserving your energy to be able to serve your body, health, and energy for your highest good.

There are a couple of remaining ways that I fine-tune being able to set myself up for success daily. I work to make sure that I don't let the yuck take over my brain. Do you know the yuck I'm talking about? I mean the sickness yuck! It's the yuck that takes over our brains and attempts to convince us that we are hopeless, helpless, a burden on society and those that we love, and are just going to continue to overall suck at life. I don't mean to sound cheesy, but it's crucial to guard against these kinds of thoughts. When you find, your mind going there remember to validate it and move on! Don't deny it, don't argue against it, don't judge it, don't evaluate it, just validate it and move on.

I work from a format of gratitude regularly. Are you ready for a mortifying story? I was reading this book all about intentional gratitude, and I was absolutely fascinated. One of the things it focused on was being grateful for EVERYTHING that happens in your life. The good, the bad, and the in-between. I made the decision that I was going to start doing this the next day. That Sunday when I woke up and was on my way to the office to start seeing clients, I noticed my head was hurting more than normal. I tried all of the normal things; caffeine, food, sleep, hypnosis, literally all the things! Before noon, I was sitting with a client, and I knew I was going to be puking soon. I was trying to get these clients out of my office and my words were beginning to slur, the sweating had started, and I KNEW that it wouldn't be long before I'd be puking. I was so very sick! Driving home I pulled over three times to puke. One of those times, a voice inside my head reminded me that today was the day I had committed to beginning to practice intentional gratitude. I thought through this process. There was no way in hell I was going to be grateful for a migraine or even puking. I mean, how does that even work?! Then it hit me! What if I was grateful for my body being able to send me such a clear message? What if I was able to be grateful for being able to have a flexible job that allows me to go home and rest? How would things shift if I could, just for a moment, experience the gratitude for being able to go home and get some rest in the middle of a migraine? I'm not going to lie to you and tell you that at that moment my migraine was removed. Because, again, that would be a miracle and I'd have my television show and be super famous! The next day, though, the weight of the world shifted just a little bit.

Whenever I get stressed, overwhelmed, or burned out one of the best ways I set myself up for success is that I begin and end with gratitude. It's been a staple in my life for as long as I can remember. Sometimes I just make a list of things, experiences, and people that I am grateful for. Oftentimes, I use the format of, I am grateful for _______________________ because _____________. When I want to take it to another level, I do some meditation and focus on the thing I am grateful for and where I feel that in my physical body and see if I can enhance that feeling or sensation.

The final way I set myself up for success daily, is to engage in either some level of meditation or self-hypnosis regularly. De-stressing your mind and body from the mental clutter and chatter of the world is super beneficial. Allowing yourself to have that reprieve from the world, and especially your illness is paramount to being successful in life and in living with an invisible illness.

CHAPTER 10

You, Alone, Determine Your Worth:

While living with chronic diseases, so many of us have allowed our self-worth to be determined by everyone and everything around us. This includes the nature, severity, and (sometimes lack) diagnoses. This is oftentimes very lethal to our mental well-being, our resilience, and our overall sense of worth as human beings. I am going to show you how important it is to declare, affirm, and be utterly and completely convinced of exactly how worthy you are. The quick and easy suggestions that I teach my clients are using affirmations, celebrating every single success (because while living with the chronic disease there are honestly lots of small little successes every single day!), stopping the deadly comparison game, changing the story, guarding your language, and doing the mirror work (seriously, I know it's super annoying, but it pays off).

Before developing a sense of self-worth, I would allow anyone to walk all over me and speak to me in absolutely unacceptable ways. I remember what happened many years ago after I had been in a massive car accident where an elderly gentleman blatantly ran a red light in the middle of a torrential downpour. I specifically remember how I went from previously having no pain in my back to excruciating pain in my lower back. It suddenly hurt to stand, walk, or move all the time. Every breathing and waking moment were filled with pain. The event that is etched in my memory is when I had an MRI done and I was reviewing the results (in an attempt to locate the pain) with this surgeon guy. To this day I can't remember his name or his specialty. I remember he spent less than five minutes with me and had a demeanor of absolute arrogance. I've since learned that if that's the doctor's baseline demeanor then they and I just won't be a good fit. This doctor flew into the room, with my MRI in hand, didn't introduce himself, and stated they couldn't get a good image as the MRI machine couldn't read me because I was so "fat". Therefore, was nothing he could do for me. He went on to say that all my problems were due to my weight. I attempted to question this logic because before the car accident I had been pain-free, but he talked all over me, discounted my experience, and sent me on my way. I felt so invalidated, invisible, and worthless. Let's be very clear, being the person, I am today if another human being (with or without a medical degree) spoke to me in the same manner that provider spoke to me, then the only reason I would be silent is that I would be afraid opening my mouth and releasing an unadulterated rage that they may not survive. I aim to act with grace and kindness most days.

When we live with chronic diseases which are all too often invisible, we frequently live with shame, regret, remorse, and self-blame. These emotions are like the four horsemen of self-worth destruction for those of us already feeling or at least living our lives being overly responsible for things such as taking up too much space, needing rest, needing guidance, needing assistance, needing assurance, needing any level of help or accommodation, and frequently losing hope. When these four horsemen are constantly beating against your self-worth, it's no wonder why it's difficult to remain intact. Many of us live in bodies that feel like we are at war with them, and they are constantly betraying us. While well-intentioned (but ill-informed) humans will mutter things like, "just don't take things personally", at us, it's next to impossible to do that when the very vessel you reside in doesn't feel safe.

Shame is another broken cog in the wheel that makes it impossible to develop a smooth system to build substantial self-worth. Shame is often seen as a very corrosive thread that slowly and systemically sucks the joy and peace out of our lives. Many people often describe shame as that feeling, emotion, sensation, or thought of not being enough and therefore unworthy of connection. To take that a step further for those of us with chronic illnesses, it typically shows up as the belief that we are not healthy enough, and therefore unworthy of connection. We are not productive enough and therefore unworthy of connection. We are not normal enough and therefore not worthy of love and connection. I could go on and on all day, but hopefully, you get the point.

When the majority of the world is made up of normal, healthy, able-bodied humans, or at a minimum created for those people to excel, it is problematic and it becomes difficult to not allow those barriers to impact your sense of self. It can be from little things like chairs with rigid arms on them for those of us larger people, to no elevators for those of us with mobility issues, to no sight options for those of us with vision problems. Let's be honest, the world is not stacked for our benefit. Don't even get me started on how many public bathrooms have mold in them. The number of times my throat has started to swell shut because of that is just too high to count.

Rather than just give you a trite and unrealistic response like, "just don't take things personally", which will likely make you want to poke my eyes out and set this book on fire, let's talk about solutions that will work. You see, I remember being that person who honestly and truly believed that everyone else's opinion was more valid and important than mine was. Currently, at this moment, there are certain issues about my own body that you will just never change my opinion about. You can show me all the research about how whatever it works for every other body on the planet. I'm still not going to buy in, because I know my body! I'm its biggest advocate!

I have likely talked about using affirmations several times in this book already. I'm passionate about affirmations. They have done so much for me in my life. From mindset work to positive thinking, to clarity and focus, including pain management, and even some healing. I rely significantly on the healing that comes through using affirmations. I also absolutely geek out about language though, which would probably make any of my Kindergarten to Twelfth-grade teachers die if they knew that. My sincerest apologies to them for my lack of dedication at the time. What I love about affirmations is that every single word in the English language has meaning. When I'm creating my affirmations, I'm very specific about the language that I'm using. It's also important to realize that our subconscious mind is action-word oriented. Just today, I was having a conversation with a client who had been waking up with 3 am thoughts that kept spiraling out of control. I asked her to walk me through what was happening. She described that as soon as she woke up to use the bathroom, she would say to herself, "I am not going to think about that issue" or "I don't want to think about that issue." I reminded her that the subconscious mind only focuses on the action words and therefore was only hearing her command to focus on the thought. She was gutted. When you are creating affirmations keep them simple, start the affirmation with the power word such as I AM, and then insert the action word with the desired outcome. Such as healing, walking, improving, etc. Honestly, I could teach a whole Master Class about affirmations. Handwritten affirmations are so much more powerful than typed ones. Handwrite them a few times a day, put them on the mirror, sing them into songs, speak to them in the mirror, make it a game and have fun with this!

Reality check for a quick second; how deeply and profoundly annoyed were you really when I suggested you begin celebrating every success? How much did you want to throw stuff at me when I dared to take that a bit too far and blatantly state that you had lots of little successes every day? Did it make you a little bit mad? Did your face get a little red? Did you slam the book shut? Did you throw it across the room? Where are we really at? As much as this concept sucks, guess what; it's still true! No matter how sick you are, no matter how far down the barrel you are, there are still successes!

Success occurs in any situation. In my adult life, I have been homeless, and I still had success. Do you know what it was? I kept a job during that chaotic and stressful time. During the height of my illness, when I was puking every day, sobbing from so much unmanageable pain, getting lost, and calling my husband crying because I couldn't find my way home, I still had success. Do you want to guess what it was? I was still alive. Some days, if that's all I have, that's okay! I'm just going to hold the hell on because I've been doing this long enough to know that the horrible storm, I'm going through is going to pass. Here's the thing, I want you to think about that last time you had a good day. Do you remember it? Do you remember what made it good? Did you feel free? Were you having fun? Did you laugh? Did you enjoy yourself? At any point during that day where you worried you were going to feel that way FOREVER? Did you have lingering and consuming feeling that you were going to have all those wonderful and happy feelings every day for the rest of your life? Odds are, no! I've been asking this question for over 25 years and never get a yes. That proves my point that no feeling, emotion, or state lasts forever. Nothing is permanent.

Create a box, a file folder, a drawer, or a folder on your computer, just make space to start collecting all of these successes. Every single day I want you to evaluate your successes. Did you get any compliments today? Was someone kind to you? Did someone go out of their way to do something nice for you? All of that needs to go into those spaces, and when you start sinking, I want you to pull out your success box and review it.

Listen, let's be honest; those people we are comparing ourselves to are not us. They are not living with our immune systems, our mental health histories, and our bodies. It's not a fair comparison so it's just a backward way of being able to beat yourself up. If you want to beat yourself up, just do it and own that. Don't utilize other people to justify beating yourself up. Most of the time, we are comparing our internal responses to what someone else projects and what we perceive about their projections. Have a look at that statement again and see how many errors and messed-up things there are about it. That's like comparing strawberries and corn, and then getting mad at the strawberries for not being on a big cob and not being yellow enough. If I presented that case to you, I suspect you would look at me like I had twelve heads and tell me that was the dumbest comparison ever. Please stop the deadly comparison game. You are freaking amazing. No one can ever compete with the amazing human being you are!

If I lived inside your brain for 24 or 48 hours, what kind of self-talk would I witness you voicing about yourself? What kind of stories do you play on repeat about yourself that either is not true or are not what you want? I've looked at research that showed that many of us do so much damage because of the story we keep repeating to ourselves. Let me ask you a question for a moment, is your internal dialogue, one of disappointment, failure, insecurity, fear, inadequacy, betrayal, or similar ideas? Then we have a huge issue and it's really in your head. Unfortunately, all the hard work you keep doing, all the therapists you have seen, and all the self-help books you read, are not going to fix it. That's because any of the work we do to rebuild or fix our self-worth is consistently destroyed because of the chatter that's happening in our heads. I mean, think about how incessant that is. Do you think the actions you've taken could compete with that? Imagine for a moment what would shift or change, and possibly improve, if you spent time every single day telling yourself positive, wonderful, and uplifting stories about yourself. It's life-altering to change the stories we tell ourselves. Make a conscious effort to begin creating new stories and focus on them. My experience, those of my friends and clients, as well as so much research all confirms that what you say to yourself reinforces who you believe yourself to be.

Guarding your language is something that typically brings a lot of controversies, but it's been a huge staple for me. It's helped so many of my clients as well. I rarely say I have "X" disease. I typically say I have been diagnosed with "X" disease. I have a friend who always says,

"I have been offered "X" diagnosis". However, as someone who works with diagnoses all day long and understands that it just means I currently meet a certain set of criteria, saying "I have been offered" doesn't feel authentic to me. The reason I don't say I have "X" disease is that I never want to take on that label or diagnosis. I have watched people for the last twenty-plus years who, once they received a diagnosis, made that part of their personality. They completely took on that entire diagnosis and made it their life. They couldn't separate it from who they were as a person. I'm acutely aware that my subconscious mind is a ginormous computer in my brain waiting for my next order. Therefore, I'm not going to write a bad program by giving it bad wording or bad language.

Here's another example of something (that again, most people don't buy into) that I'm diligent about. I don't ever use the word lose in the context of weight. So many people have a psychological tie between losing and finding, and that applies to weight as well. When they say the word 'lose', their subconscious mindsets out to find it. Don't believe me? Cool! Let me demonstrate. How do you react when you lose your house keys, car keys, wallet, debit card, cell phone, or anything else of importance? How much do you freak out!? How determined are you to find it? Depending on your response to losing things, that is exactly how psychological ties are created. So, when we are all walking around talking about how we lost 5 pounds, then our subconscious mindsets out to find it for us. BOOM randomly one day it magically reappears. It's very cyclical! There are so many examples of this.

I'm not going to lie to you, I don't think anyone with a chronic disease or illness LOVES mirror work! I mean, at the height of my disease I had mastered the delicate art of being able to look in a full-length mirror and only see my hair and teeth. It was a very skillful process, honestly! However, every time I passed the mirror it triggered the release of this negative diatribe in my brain in which I berated myself and talked to myself as if I was the worst person on the planet. So, yeah, it's going to be uncomfortable. It's going to feel very unsettling. Start really simple. In the beginning, I want you to get as close as you can to the mirror, just look at your eyes. Only your eyes! Stare deep into your eyes, and first thing in the morning tell your eyes, "Good morning Gorgeous, Have a great day!" At lunch, go back to looking deep into your eyes, so deep that you can't see anything else, and just tell yourself, "Hey there friend, you are rocking things today." Then at bedtime, repeat the same process and just tell yourself, "Good night, because I love you." As you get more and more comfortable with this mirror work, you can pull a little farther away and bring more of yourself into view. Remember to go super slow, I don't want you to become dysregulated and feel unsafe. Once you are finally able to fully see yourself in the mirror, begin repeating affirmations out loud in the mirror. Eventually, the goal is just to affirm how much value that amazingly awesome person in the mirror has!

CHAPTER 11

Making It All Work

Together we've covered so much content here. Honestly, if we were sitting down and talking over coffee, they would have probably closed the coffee shop so many times and reopened it that they would have demanded we pay rent by now. To say I have a ton of information in my brain and am trying not to overwhelm you with how to apply it would be the understatement of the century. Therefore, I'd like to spend a little time outlining, in a general sense, what a practical application looks like.

I'm going to, to be honest with you, I may have a wee bit of a book buying obsession. I love the idea of a brand-new book. I love the concept of sitting down, setting time aside, and diving into a new book. However, here's the thing, I rarely ever finish most of these books. Lots of people believe that it's because I have gotten what I needed from those books, blah, blah, blah. Can I tell you a huge secret, though? Some of those books I'm not even sure I read. I don't want that to be your experience when you read this book! I want you to walk away from this book feeling empowered, re-energized, hopeful, and confident. I want you to know, beyond a shadow of a doubt, and with the utmost conviction, that you know how to apply the knowledge we've looked at in this book.

Remember how I shared with you that I was taking naps between clients, using a wheelchair to get into the office, and many days puking before and after clients from migraines? It was absolutely brutal, honesty! If we go back through this book, I was living my life in a CRAMMED manner. Oof, and it was so brutal too, let me tell you. I was constantly confused about what I was doing, where I was supposed to be, where I was going, what medication or supplement I was supposed to be taking, and just so much else. In a sincere effort to see improvement, I spent countless hours down endless rabbit holes. I had a deep level of repressed anger about being sick, having been misdiagnosed and undiagnosed for so very long, and not feeling seen by the medical community. The constant misdirection that I experienced from multiple medical providers didn't help anything. One provider would contradict another provider who would yet still contradict a third provider. It was maddening. I experienced deepening levels of mistrust towards my own body, towards the medical community, and towards the world that doesn't enforce better screenings of these diseases. I can't begin to describe the depth of the well of evasion I was in. I evaded everything and everyone that got too close because they might ask something and expect more than a superficial answer. To be honest, it was a toss-up that scared me worse; the thought of breaking someone else with the truth of how sick and in pain I was, or the thought of breaking myself with those admissions. Every molecule of my being and every moment of my life was filled with despair. I think it clouded every interaction, every relationship, and every moment I engaged with someone. This may sound a bit harsh and trust me, I have all the compassion in the world for the struggles you may be going through, however, it's impossible to focus on healing and improving your mind and body when you are stuck in that CRAMMED state. Does that make sense?

When I made the decision that I didn't want the diseases to rule my life anymore, I recognized that I needed to take control of my life again, otherwise it was going to rot my brain. I had to make the conscious switch to begin focusing on, developing, and embracing a CHARMED lifestyle. It was not easy at first, and honestly, I kept getting caught up in the fact that I didn't believe it was true. To be honest, I worked to hold onto this the way you hold to jello. Have you ever tried to hold jello? The tighter you hold onto it the more it slips through your fingers. Initially, I started by writing CHARMED on my mirror and each day I would take a few minutes and set my intention to focus on one of the words. Each day, during the day, I would take a few moments and focus on ways to increase the sensations and experiences of each of those words. It enhanced my ability to notice the experiences and opportunities for each of those words and sensations.

I literally cannot write enough about the power of validation. It's been so important, not just in my life, but in the lives of my clients, friends, family members, etc. I spend at least three sessions per day talking to clients about it. I keep stressing it, even if I have talked to the clients, I'm working with five million times before because sometimes we all need reminders about things. That's okay because I will give all the reminders necessary in the world. The biggest struggle for me personally was that no one warned me about the grief aspect. I grieved so hard for the normalcy that I longed for and I kept trying to pretend like I was just "happy" in this chronically unwell body. It wasn't working for me, though! I forced myself to get real and honest with myself and just acknowledge that living in a chronically unwell body with a bunch of different diseases sucked. There was no cure for them, but I could hope for remission, and I could validate that, yep, this sucked massively! As long as I didn't take up permanent residence there and have my mail forwarded there, I didn't have a problem with it. In honoring and validating that, yes, my experience sucked, what I found was that the feeling and sensation lessened. I was able to move on. It can be as simple as validating our current experiences and switching our focus to something opposite. I tend to switch my focus to gratitude or something that I love. You have to find what works for you, though.

Learning how to advocate, for me, was honestly one of the more difficult concepts to apply myself. Depending on your background and prior experiences this may be a particular area of struggle for you as well. Me, in the beginning, I had no idea what it could be like to advocate for myself, what that looked like, or even how it worked. I'm not sure how it works for the average person, so I'm just going to tell you what I did. I watched people, and I mean I watched lots of people. I observed so many people in general, and then I focused on the people who did a stellar job of advocating for themselves or others. I began by using that as a script in my brain. In the beginning, I would mimic the exact words that they said. Oftentimes, I simply inserted my name or a slight change in the script that I'd heard them say. Once I gave it a shot and had a couple of times where I experienced successes, my desire to advocate for myself spread like wildfire.

Sorting your way through boundary development is like building a house blindfolded. This is particularly so if you grew up in a house like I did where it was never a conversation. I began exploring how I felt in my relationships. Not just in my marriage or with my closest friends, but in my relationships with my clients, with my employees, with my providers, with my children, with my neighbors, with my in-laws, with my acquaintances, and with everyone I interacted with. As I was evaluating these relationships, I examined them to see if these relationships were fulfilling, if they nurtured my soul, if they were draining, how they made me feel about myself, etc. Then, depending on how those answers came back, I may or may not have dug a bit deeper or put firmer or looser boundaries in place.

I truly believe that everything I've already discussed laid the solid foundation for how to develop the conviction and belief that what you are experiencing is your sense of normalcy. For me, it was the internal conviction that something was normal or not because I said so. Now don't get me wrong, there are still times I honestly don't know, which is why I have installed human pillars to act as reality/normalcy barometers. These are the sacred people who I can send a picture of a mole and be like, "does this look normal", or a massive infection on my body that's disgusting, I can text or message them and tell them I think I'm from an alternate planet because of all these remarkable reasons. I can tell them about these stabbing or burning sensations, and we can talk through if these are normal or not. Specifically, if you don't have that internal locus of control regarding what is normal and what is not normal it's a good idea to have people in your life who can support you unconditionally and who have your best interest at heart.

When you begin personalizing your plan, and setting yourself up for success daily, remember that what works for me may not work for you. That's okay, though, don't beat yourself up about it. Adapt it in a way that works for you and move on. I do. Everyone I know who takes medications swears by establishing their medications in a pill container a week/month at a time. Here's why that just doesn't work for me, though; many of my medications don't get taken at the house. Even of those that do, I lose a few weeks once the container runs out of pills. What works better for me is to put the pills in snack-size zip-lock baggies. My friends who are closest to me laugh because I'm famous for having a zip lock baggie of pills in my purse. The point is, that I'm constantly evaluating ways to set myself up for success. I'm always looking at what's working and what's not working, what I can tweak to improve or enhance, as well as what I need to back off on to help me more effectively. Start with something small and build from there. Don't attempt to scale the whole mountain at once, especially if you haven't even been walking recently.

When I first received my initial diagnosis, my self-worth probably couldn't have gotten any lower. Since then, I have done a ton of work to be able to be the main person who sets my worth. Unless someone is in my inner circle, their opinion doesn't carry any weight or validity toward my worth. Because trust me, people will have all kinds of opinions about your disease, illness, healing, recovery, and the way you live your life. Not only that, they will freely give you their opinion at every opportunity! I created a safe space in my house that's just mine, even my husband isn't allowed in there without me. However ridiculous it sounds, it's a room that we painted about 9 shades to get the correct shade with the appropriate glitter-to-paint ratio. I call it my Zen Den and even the dog is only allowed in there when I'm in there with her. The room has cool lighting that I love as well. I make it a goal to spend a bit of time in there on most nights. Some evenings it's just fifteen minutes and other nights it's a few hours. My husband has even commented at this point on how much more relaxed I am when I spend time there versus when I don't. When I'm in my Zen Den, I use my cool pen and my special journal, and I focus on doing some handwritten journaling. I handwrite out my affirmations. I do some future scripted journaling to help program my subconscious mind for success.

Please don't misunderstand me, it is true that none of this will cure or reduce your disease or pain! That's unrealistic and I would just be flat-out lying if I attempted to try and spew that kind of garbage. I'm just not willing to have my ethics challenged or questioned in that manner. Having said that, let me tell you about my friend, Sally. Sally continued to struggle with finding an accurate diagnosis for five years. As a good friend, I continued to attempt to empower her to get an accurate diagnosis, but it never created any change for her. However, once I started walking Sally through the philosophies outlined in this book, she was able to advocate for herself. She finally gained an official diagnosis, and a solid treatment plan, and was able to get her head into moving forward. She began setting herself up for success, and slowly but surely advocating for herself. Eventually, she stopped questioning every single thing, and believing doctors when they would blow her off, and started standing up for herself. She was like a different person!

If you want these same changes in your life, just follow the steps outlined in this book. Break it down into manageable steps and adapt it to work for you. Remember that if it doesn't currently apply to you, pause it and revisit it later, because what doesn't apply right here right now may apply later, or may apply differently on a different day.

I hope this book brings you so much peace and takes your healing journey to another level!

CHAPTER 12

Parting Thoughts

Many of us with chronic disease, chronic illnesses, and chronic pain tend toward all-or-nothing tendencies. I can't tell you how many of the clients I work with who have chronic diseases and will either do all of the thing's doctors, experts, therapists, etc. recommend or they will do absolutely nothing! I have watched it countless times and it baffles my brain every time. I just don't understand the mentality, it feels like abandoning your ship in the middle of the ocean and then later getting mad because your ship is all damaged and battered. But you are the one that abandoned the ship, remember? Yet, when I want to walk away from everything and go to Tahiti, I'm engaging in the same thing. I recommend making a list of your non-negotiables. These are the things that you will do day in and day out no matter what. For me, every single day, no matter what, I'm going to take my thyroid medication because I have no thyroid. That's non-negotiable, no matter what. There are certain medications and supplements that I work painstakingly to ensure that I don't run out of because not taking them is not an option for me.

Again, I understand how overwhelming it is to live with chronic diseases, chronic illnesses, and chronic pain. Many times, we are bouncing around from provider to provider none of whom can make up their mind on a diagnosis, and it regularly feels like people with medical degrees are just throwing sludge at the wall hoping against hope that something, anything, sticks and maybe something will work. I don't think healthy able-bodied people can understand the devastating hopelessness that these experiences spawn. Specifically, few people seem aware of the scarring amount of shame that these experiences create. When you are drowning in medical appointments, well-intentioned people who are bombarding you with all of the opinions, random strangers off the street verbally bombing you with their ill-informed opinions as if they were medical experts, all while attempting to do your research, it's near impossible to keep your head above water! My parting words to you are to help you develop a scheme where you can navigate making this book work for you.

Make a written list of the things that you are committing to as you commit to them. Make a checklist to keep you committed to the process. If you have any level of brain fog, you are going to forget, and then you will backslide, and you will regress exponentially. You don't want that, and I don't want that for you! Track as much as possible, whether that's in writing or on apps on your phone. Learn how to keep lists, use apps, and stop relying on your amazing brain. While it is amazing, it's not infallible. I think we covered a concept somewhere about setting ourselves up for success, didn't we?

Create an accountability or support group. Talk to loved ones about key concepts that you got from this group. Share insights and highlights with loved ones and trusted family members. Sharing these things will help keep you accountable. When we share things with the important people in our lives and allow them in, they can help hold us accountable. They also get a glimpse of what we struggle with, as well as what our perceived weaknesses are. Having accountability and support will ensure that you are more empowered and likely more successful in implementing the suggestions in this book.

Understand that you will likely benefit from reading this book more than once. Most of the books that changed my life or positively influenced my life I keep going back to, reading them over and over again. The same goes for those life-altering movies. There are movies I watch when I need to strengthen my faith, ones I watch when I need a good soul-cleansing cry and ones I watch when I need a deep laugh. Books are the same. Please be prepared to read this book several times. There are so many deep nuances in this book, you are likely to have missed some of them the first time through. Plan on reading this book a few times at minimum to grasp the depth and significance of everything that's packed in this book. You deserve that.

Surround yourself with bursts of inspiration. It doesn't have to be affirmations; you can use quotes from people who you find inspirational. It can be thank you card for something nice or kind you did for someone else. It can be a picture of people who are part of what keeps pushing you to put one foot in front of the other. It can be destination pictures of places you will go when your health improves or whatever your long-term goal is. The list is endless, and it really depends on what works for you.

Identify and focus on your why. I'm sure you have heard this countless times already, and by now it's probably begun to sound trite. However, it does have a significant amount of validity. Getting down to the source of your why is really about understanding and knowing why you keep pushing forward. Identify what motivates you and use that to help continue to propel yourself and maximize your momentum. Not knowing or understanding our why oftentimes leaves us wandering in the middle of the desert. For a long time, my focus was on reducing the massive pain I experienced. Later it was to increase my energy because it felt like my energy was consistently massively depleted. Later on in my journey, the focus became attempting to reduce the inflammation my body carries which I measured by the amount of weight my body holds. I always know what I'm focused on and what I'm working towards. If you don't know what you are working towards, how do you measure success? To me, that feels like being stuck in a holding pattern. When you are living with chronic disease things are already frustrating and maddening enough without adding hanging out in a holding pattern into the mix.

Remember that we are all different and you have to find a way to make this work for you. Don't allow yourself to get caught up in what works for someone else, including me, or not being good enough, or whatever else. Please also heed this very crucial warning; you will need to do the emotional work alongside having a chronic illness. Remember that there's a high correlation between chronic disease and depression. Don't be so proud that you attempt to just shove that into a tiny box and think you can manage it all by yourself. That's just a deadly level of pride that is not going to help you or serve you well.

Whatever else you do, don't you dare ever give up! It doesn't matter how bad things get, it doesn't matter how sick you feel, it doesn't matter what diagnosis they toss at you, don't you dare give up! You are better than that, you deserve more than that, and you had better not settle for anything less. Even if you have to work to apply these things five million times until they work for you, keep doing it. Just like everything else in life, hard work always pays off, but it's continuing to put one foot in front of the other that is the struggle for many of us.

My final thought as our time together comes to a close, is this; I would love for you to spend some time meditating on what you are thinking, spending time engaging in, doing, etc., and how these things are promoting your healing. Another thing to spend time doing is to just meditate and ask yourself how to promote your healing, how to take it to the next step, and so on. One of the best things I do regularly ask myself, "How does this promote my healing"? In my experience, maintaining this level of focus helps me to guard against getting sucked into the negativity and cesspool of being sick, being in pain, being miserable, and on and on the list goes!

Don't forget how amazing you truly are!

"It takes a ton of courage to wake up every day and face the world again and again."

Living with a chronic illness often comes with feelings of pain, hopelessness, fear, and anxiety. It is debilitating to constantly live in a body that feels like it's betraying you. Jenn Bovee, a licensed psychotherapist and manager of her own chronic illness, offers a refreshing, empathetic perspective on how to thrive with a chronic illness.

Written with a touch of humor, personal stories, and practical advice, this book teaches you how to advocate for yourself, to use your voice, and to use validation so you are living a life where you aren't ashamed to take up space.

www.ingramcontent.com/pod-product-compliance
Lightning Source LLC
Chambersburg PA
CBHW021112130726
47988CB00003B/987